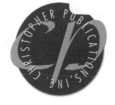

Dr. Christopher's
Guide To
Colon Health

Formally, Rejuvenation Through Elimination
By Dr. John R. Christopher, M.H., N.D.

Supervising Editor: David Christopher M.H. A.H.G.
Contributing Editor: Nathan Jaynes M.H.
Cover design by Reid Johns
Herb drawings by Kaye Thorne
Anatomy illustrations by Nathan Jaynes M.H.

Copyright 1976 by John R. Christopher
Revised and expanded 2003
ISBN# 1-879436-20-5

Disclaimer:
The information presented in this book is for educational purposes only and
is not meant to take the place of diagnosis and treatment by a qualified
health care provider.

Table of Contents

Who's In Charge?

All the organs of the body were having a meeting, trying to decide who was the one in charge.

"I should be in charge," said the brain "because I run all the body's systems, so without me nothing would happen."

"I should be in charge," said the blood "because I circulate oxygen all over, so without me you'd all waste away."

"I should be in charge," said the stomach "because I process food and give all of you energy."

"I should be in charge," said the legs "because I carry the body wherever it needs to go."

"I should be in charge," said the eyes "because I allow the body to see where it is going."

" I should be in charge," said the bowel "because I'm responsible for waste removal."

All the other body parts laughed at the bowel and insulted him, so in a huff, he shut down tight. Within a few days, the brain had a terrible headache, the stomach was bloated, the legs got wobbly, the eyes got watery, and the blood became toxic. All the organs decided the bowel should be the boss. The moral of the story? Some bum is usually in charge.

Introduction

When my father first wrote this work, it was a small booklet designed to be a quick reference guide for anyone interested in intestinal health. It gave basic instructions on how to maintain a healthy colon and what to do for gastrointestinal diseases. Over the years many people have wanted a more detailed description of what herbs to use for specific diseases and a step by step approach to bowel cleansing. I have no doubt that if Dr. Christopher were living now he would be updating and revising his work to include this information.

One of the challenges of updating someone else's work is trying to follow the same philosophy and style. Dr. Christopher liked to keep things simple and natural. He sought to empower his students and readers so they could heal themselves without having to rely on doctors, medicines, or machines. Besides being known as a wonderful teacher, Dr. Christopher was also a great learner. He loved and respected the work of the great healers of the past as well as his peers including Hypocrates, Samuel Thompson, Dr. John Harvey Kellogg, Dr. Nowell, and Norman W. Walker. Dr. Christopher quoted some of these men in his original text, and this new edition continues to honor their timeless work. We hope you enjoy the historical flavor of these writings as well as the additional information included.

I would like to give a special thanks to Nathan Jaynes, Tara and Jerem Eyre, Lindsay Wolsey, and Cheryl Vose, in the "rejuvenation" of this valuable work.

David Christopher M.H., A.H.G.

Forward

S tart any conversation with an herbalist and sooner or later they'll start talking about the Colon. Whether the topic turns to chronic constipation or diverticulitis, countless lunches have been ruined by talkative herbalists. Why the fascination with the intestines? Natural healers realize that nine out of ten diseases are caused by constipation and can be prevented and treated with a proper diet and herbal formulas. In an ideal world, everyone would have three bowel movements a day, wholesome food would be the norm rather than the exception, disease would be uncommon, and herbalists would have very little to talk about.

The intestines may not be a topic of polite conversation, but maybe they should be. The social stigma associated with discussing anything remotely bowel oriented is causing millions of people to suffer silently with their diseases. It is estimated that as many as one million people are currently living with inflammatory bowel disease in America. Twenty percent of the population experiences some form of irritable bowel syndrome. Diverticular disease affects approximately two million people and each year three hundred thousand new cases of diverticulitis are diagnosed. These conditions are often ignored by the media which would rather talk about anything else.

Natural healers have recognized the connection between the colon and health for centuries. The Hindu Vedas, which are the oldest known medical texts, described both enema and laxative use more than four thousand years ago. The ancient Egyptians were also concerned about bowel health. The Ebers Papyrus (an Egyptian medical document written three thousand years ago) describes bowel health, and details what to do for several bowel conditions. In these writings the Egyptians catalogued many laxative herbs, used to clean the colon. Hypocrates, the famous Greek doctor and the "Father of

Medicine" (460 BC), left behind many writings that were used as medical text books for centuries and are still used today. He referred to various ways of cleaning the intestines and described using a bull's horn or a pig's bladder and a hollow reed or cane to administer an enema. The Essenes who lived during the times of the New Testament also wrote about bowel health, one of the Essene gospels states that "The uncleanness within is greater than the uncleanness without. And he who cleanses himself without, but within remains unclean, is like a tomb that outward is painted fair, but is within full of all manner of horrible uncleanliness and abominations." The Essenes strongly believed in using herbs to maintain colon health.

This tradition of internal cleansing has been passed down from generation to generation of natural healers. Dr. John Harvey Kellogg (of Kellogg's Corn Flake fame), ran a sanitarium where he treated thousands of people for many different ailments. Dr. Kellogg reported in the 1917 *Journal of American Medicine* that out of over 40,000 cases of gastrointestinal disease, he had used surgery only twenty times. The rest were helped as a result of cleansing the bowels, diet and exercise. He also published a comprehensive book on colon hydrotherapy and the bowel's effect on health. Jethro Kloss (who practiced natural healing in the 1920s) wrote about the importance of fasting, a plant based diet, and internal cleansing. Dr. Nowell (one of Dr. Christopher's instructors) also taught about the connection between intestinal health and the rest of the body. Bernard Jensen D.C. and Iridologist taught colon health in his lectures and books, he wrote "In times past, knowledge of the bowel was more widespread and people were taught how to care for the bowel. Somehow, bowel wisdom got lost and it became something that no one wanted to talk about anymore." Dr. Christopher also felt strongly about colon health and proper diet. His focus on intestinal health has saved thousands of people who would have otherwise suffered needlessly.

Modern herbalists should have just as much, if not more concern about colon health than their earlier predecessors.

Healers of old didn't have to worry about today's epidemics of obesity, bowel disease, and cancer because ancient people didn't have fast food, carbonated beverages, and office jobs that create these problems. Today's society needs to come to terms with their bowel instead of ignoring it like some dirty secret. Hopefully one day the lowly bowel will once again find its way back into polite conversation. Maybe then more herbalists will get invited to lunch.

Nathan Jaynes M.H., Editor

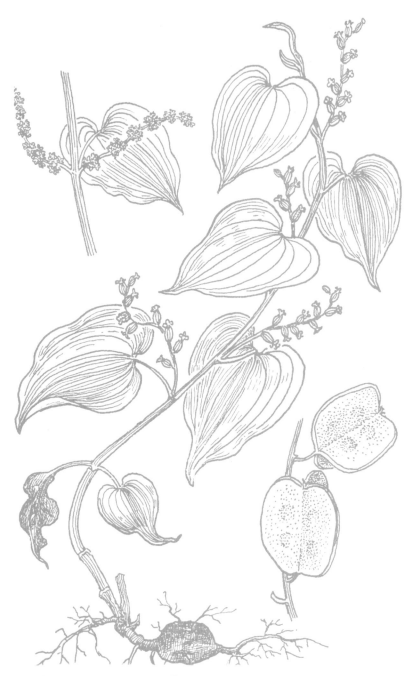

> "To eat is human.
> To digest, divine."
> —Mark Twain

Chapter 1

The Digestive System

Our bodies must be kept clean, inside and out, to perform their tasks efficiently and smoothly. The body is the housing of the spirit, the operating force of life. With the spirit commanding a good clean structure—smoother, happier lives will result. We have been told scripturally that our body is a temple, or tabernacle of God, and God will not dwell in an unclean tabernacle. So we must keep our bodies clean and in good repair for them to be comfortable abodes.

As we stand in small close areas with other people, their body odors can tell us a lot about their internal condition. The strong odor or fumes from alcoholic beverages emanate from the body and can be very repulsive. A constipated person also has a hard time covering his or her offensive body odor and uses deodorants and perfumes to disguise this unsavory condition.

We can compare this bad body odor caused by constipation to opening the door to our home after an extended absence and being greeted by the staggering foul odor of a backed up sewer. There are two ways this nauseating odor can be eliminated. One way is to cover the effect by buying room fresheners and spraying the area to neutralize the disagreeable scent. Reoccurrence is assured and the stench will return because this is only a temporary fix, nothing has been done about the cause of the smell. The wiser way is to remove the cause by unplugging and cleaning out the sewer line so there will be no more backing up of sewage.

Many of us have a sewage line that is backed up or constipated, and the horrible odor of halitosis comes out our front door (the mouth) as it is opened. Someone says, "Your breath is horrible," so most of us work on just the effect by popping in a mint or running for the mouthwash to cover our bad breath. If someone says, "Whew—you need a bath; the smell of your body is awful," most of us again work only on the effect and use underarm deodorant, perfumes, colognes, etc. We never think of cleaning up the cause, which not only affects how we smell, but our health.

Well over ninety percent of all disease comes from an unclean body whose sewer is backed up. A backed-up sewer means our filth has accumulated throughout the body. When this happens, you are dirty and filthy inside, the body does not operate as well, and mental processes often dwell on lower thoughts and ideas rather than on a higher plane.

Our human mechanism is like a car loaded with carbon and sludge, the timing is off, the electrical system is shorting, and is badly in need of a tune-up and overhaul. By grinding the valves, cleaning out the sludge in the oil system, tuning up the poorly functioning parts of the car, it will again run as good as new. Cleaning out our vehicles (our bodies) and getting a tune-up is the most important thing we can do to have a smoothly operating body that will use less fuel (food) and get better mileage and performance.

For this to happen we need to look at the bowel. Our bowels are the most neglected and ignored parts of our bodies. We need to know how this eliminative organ works so the large intestines can be kept clean and operate as desired and intended by the original creator of our bodies.

Inherent weaknesses are often handed down from generation to generation and it is our job to rebuild, renew and improve the (dietary and lifestyle) sins of our parents and pass on better habits to future generations. Because of improper eating and not taking care of our bodies, these weaknesses get handed down to our posterity. These could be sins of omission or sins of commission. Let's change the tide and build a better body so our offspring and the generations to come will become a stronger, happier and a more peaceful race of people.

Never will we have peace as long as we have constipated warriors sitting around the peace table glaring in hate at

10

each other. Peace will come from clean, sweet, happy bodies and those who teach this natural lifestyle to their families through their example. These teachings can eventually spread worldwide.

The first steps to having a smooth-running, happy, efficient body is to first give it a three day juice cleanse and then start the mucusless diet as explained in *Dr. Christopher's Three Day Cleansing Program, Mucusless Diet, and Herbal Combinations*. This will start working on the cause of the malfunctions in the body, renewing the flesh and rebuilding organs. By continuing with this program, you are guaranteed to not have the problems of constipation and ill health any more during your life.

As we proceed along the line of the mucusless diet, do not panic for fear that you will starve. You will eat less, but you will have more vitality, less sickness, and your natural weight will be attained.

A good meal of a baked potato (if grown organically eat skin and all) or a steamed one with vegetable or olive oil, coarse freshly ground pepper and, if desired, chives and/or other condiment herbs for enhancing the flavor, along with a large vegetable salad, some steamed or low heated vegetables, fresh vegetable juice, a casserole of presoaked, low heated grains as a base (described in the above mentioned booklet— see also *Regenerative Diet* by Dr. Christopher and *Transfiguration Diet*) and you will be satisfied, without that uncomfortable bloat or hidden hunger. You will be satisfied with less food without sluggishness. With this type of diet, you will eat approximately one-third of what you eat now, have more pep and energy, as well as free, easy bowel movements. This will not happen the first day but with the help of herbal aids to tone up the bowel area plus the diet and additional items we will tell you about, you will find new life!

A must for good health is to slow down the eating procedure. Relax and be happy while you eat. Discuss pleasant things during mealtime. Laugh a little and remember the old adage of "a crust of bread with love is better than a banquet in contention." Chew each mouthful thoroughly, whether juice or solid food. Saliva is the key that opens the door to digestion. Without saliva mixed thoroughly with food or juice, the material goes down to the stomach and does not aid the gastric juices as Nature intended, causing much of the meal to be eliminated without proper assimilation.

How Digestion Works

Most people think that the digestive process begins when food enters the mouth. In reality, digestion starts in the brain, when we think about food, smell food, and see the food before we eat it. The brain sends signals around the body to prepare it for the incoming meal or snack. The brain increases salivation, production of digestive enzymes in the stomach, and makes us feel hungry. When this occurs, the body is ready to begin breaking down the food. For this to happen, our foods must be successfully processed through three important digestive areas or "mixing bowls." When any one of these areas is malfunctioning or is not properly utilized, disease often occurs. For, as Deschauer wisely asserted, "We live, not by what we eat, but by what we digest, absorb, and assimilate." It is interesting to note that as we eat, food stays outside of our bodies. The alimentary canal is like a tube with the mouth at one opening and the rectum at the other opening. Food passes through this tube and our bodies digest nutrients which are taken in or assimilated. What is not needed by the body passes through the tube and never enters the body.

The Mouth and Esophagus

The first digestive mixing bowl is the mouth, the teeth, and the salivary glands. Here, food is (or should be) ground up finely using teeth as "grinders" and mixed well with the slightly alkaline juices and enzymes of saliva that are so necessary for preparing the starches for digestion.

The body's three pairs of salivary glands are the parotid glands, the submaxillary glands, and the sublingual glands. The parotid glands are the largest and are located in front of

The Digestive System

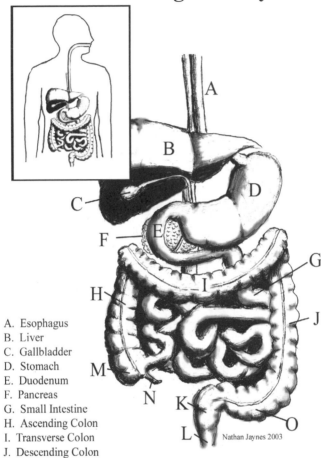

A. Esophagus
B. Liver
C. Gallbladder
D. Stomach
E. Duodenum
F. Pancreas
G. Small Intestine
H. Ascending Colon
I. Transverse Colon
J. Descending Colon
K. Rectum
L. Anus
M. Cecum
N. Vermiform Appendix
O. Sigmoid Colon

Nathan Jaynes 2003

and below the ear. The ducts of these glands open into the mouth through the cheek just opposite the second molar teeth of the upper jaw. The submaxillary glands are about the size of walnuts and are located on each side beneath the lower jaw. Their ducts open into the mouth just under the tip of the tongue. The sublingual glands are located in the floor of the mouth forming small ridges between the tongue and the gums of the lower jaw and have many ducts (some of which connect with the submaxillary glands). Between one and two pints of saliva is secreted daily into the mouth. This saliva contains, mucus, water, antibacterial proteins and salivary amylase, which converts starches into sugar. Saliva's alkaline action is important in neutralizing acids, it also moistens and softens food for passage through the esophagus.

The rate of saliva secretion depends upon what is in the mouth. Although sucking on a button or a pebble will weakly stimulate saliva flow, there are certain savory and non-savory agents called *sialogogues* which more strongly activate the salivary glands. Some herbal sialogogues include: betel leaves, blue flag root, cayenne, European elder bark, false sweet flag root, ginger root, hydrangea root, jaborandi root, lemon, and snake root.

The Stomach

When food is swallowed, it passes through the peristaltic action of the esophagus into the second digestive mixing bowl (the stomach) where gastric juices are secreted. Gastric secretions include mucus, pepsin, rennin, hydrochloric acid, hormones and intrinsic factor. The hydrochloric acid dissolves the proteins and turns food into a semifluid substance called *chyme*. The stomach is capable of considerable capacity and the motions of its muscular action serve to knead and mix the gastric juices with the processing food. It has been estimated that there are some ten to twenty pints of gastric juices secreted during a twenty-four hour period. These juices restrict the action of saliva upon the starches while in the stomach and also affect the digestion of fats. The stomach normally completes

Summary Of The Digestive Process

Site of Digestion	Glands Involved	Secretion	Enzymes	Digestive Activity
Mouth	Parotid Submaxillary Sublingual	Saliva	Salivary Amylase	Digests Starch
Esophagus	Mucus	Mucus		Lubrication
Stomach	Gastric	Gastric	Pepsin Rennin Hydrochloric Acid	Digests Protein Digests Casein Activates Pepsinogen and Kills Microorgansims
Small Intestines	Liver	Bile		Emulsifies Fats
	Pancreas	Pancreatic Juices	Amylase Lipase Peptidase	Digests Sugar Digests Fats Digests Protein
	Intestinal	Intestinal	Peptidase Sucrase Lipase Amylase Nuclease	Digests protein Digests Sugar Digests Fats Digests Sugar Digests Nucleic Acids
Large Intestines	Mucus	Mucus		Lubrication and Absorption of Nutrients

its digestive action and is emptied of its contents every four or five hours.

Agents that are specific aids in giving strength and tone to the stomach are called *stomachios* or *digestives*. Herbal digestives include agrimony, allspice, angelica, avens, bay leaves, betel leaves, thistle, chamomile, caraway seed, cardamon seed, casparilla, cayenne, condurango, coriander, dandelion root, fennel seed, gentian, horsemint, lovage, nutmeg, peppermint, pimento, quassia, sweet flag, true unicorn root, turkey rhubarb, and white cedar leaves. Food is liquefied during the digestive processes in the stomach into chyme and is gradually expelled through the pylorus (at the bottom of the stomach) into the duodenum.

The Small and Large Intestines

Almost immediately upon entering the duodenum, the chyme becomes mingled with pancreatic juices and bile and other intestinal secretions. The pancreas is a compound endocrine/exocrine gland, producing both insulin to metabolize sugar and digestive enzymes that digest fats, carbohydrates, and proteins. The pancreas is located behind the stomach with its head at the curve of the duodenum. Bile is a golden-green fluid secreted by the liver. The liver weighs around sixty ounces (the largest gland in the body) and lies under the diaphragm and over the right kidney, along the upper portion of the ascending colon, and the pyloric end of the stomach.

During digestion in the intestines, both bile and pancreatic juices enter the duodenum about three inches below the pyloric valve through the common bile duct. When digestion is in progress, the duct carries the bile into the gall bladder, which is pear shaped and located in the tissue on the underside of the liver. When the duct becomes obstructed, the bile is absorbed into the blood and gives rise to a jaundiced condition in the tissues of the body. The bile is an alkaline agent which aids pancreatic juices in digestion, prevents fermentation in the intestines, emulsifies fats, is a natural laxative, and stimulates the peristaltic action.

The healing agents that strengthen, tone and act upon the liver are *hepatic tonics* (herbs such as barberry, balimony, culver's root, dandelion, liverwort, Indian apple root, mandrake, marsh watercress, wahoo, wild yam, and wormwood). Agents that promote the flow of bile by contracting the bile ducts, but not necessarily influencing or increasing the secretion of bile, are called *cholagogues* (herbal cholagogues include aloe gum, butternut bark, culver's root, and wahoo bark).

When this third mixing is completed, the vital and regenerative elements are ready to be absorbed into the blood through the intestinal villi which take the life-giving materials into the bloodstream much like the root systems of plants assimilate necessary elements from the soil.

Dr. Nowell clearly describes this digestive function and action which takes place within the intestinal tract, as follows:

"Both the large and small intestines consist of four layers similar to the stomach. The mucus membrane forms the inner surface of the small intestine which has many small folds named Valvulae Conniventes. These folds increase the area of the secreting surface. They also prevent food from passing too quickly through the intestines, thereby allowing full opportunity for the digestive juices to do their work.

The inner surface of the small intestine is covered with a multitude of fine hairlike tubes called villi. These villi absorb nutritious matter from the food in the intestinal tract.

The mucus coat for both the large and small intestines is well supplied with glands. The glands vary, some are tubular, some are globular (Peyer's Glands), some of these are single, others are in groups (Peyer's patches). There are also others called Brunner's glands. These glands pour secretion into the intestine. In view of the many villi and glands, the student will realize how necessary it is to keep the alimentary canal clean, that the value of the food may be conveyed to the bloodstream. It is undoubtedly true that by far the greatest majority of people seeking help when sick have allowed the intestinal tract to become clogged. This will upset the whole of the organism in one form or another.

From what has been said, it will be evident that the process of digestion continues through the small intestines. It does not, however, end there. The food passes through the small intestines into the large intestine through the cecum. The cecum becomes filled, the ileocecal valve closes and the walls of the cecum contract forcing the food into the ascending colon. The motions of the intestines are called peristaltic. They are wavelike. A peculiar feature of the motions of the ascending colon is that they are called antiperistaltic. This is because they pass both ways, i.e. away from the small intestines and toward them. This keeps the food moving back and forth and delays its passage. This gives time for the absorption of materials from the food.

Owing to the absorption of soluble materials from the food in its passage through the intestines, it becomes more solid or firm, until it becomes a mass suitable for ejection. This matter is called feces.

Feces consist of undigested foods, products of decomposition, bile, and other secretions. The color of the feces is primarily caused by the pigments from the bile. In jaundice, the stools are a light, clay color, showing that the bile is not flowing.

Defecation is the name given to the ejection of feces from the anus. The anus is the outer end of the rectum. Two strong muscles guard the anal canal—the inner and outer sphincter muscles. The rectum is empty until just before defecation. Nerve stimuli produces peristaltic action in the colon using a small quantity of feces to enter the rectum. This arouses sensory nerves which bring about the desire to defecate. The rectum should be empty under normal conditions until just previous to defecation.

It is unwise to put off defecation once the desire has arisen. The small portion of feces which enter the rectum bringing the desire to defecate will, when held there, become harder. Moreover, the presence of this in the rectum causes a dulling of the sensory nerves, thereby blunting the desire to defecate. This no doubt has much to do with causing constipation in many cases. Always respond to the call of nature as soon as possible."

What is normal?

Gastrointestinal textbooks describe a normal bowel movement as a solid mass of formed fecal matter. They also state that it is normal to have one bowel movement a day or three a week. This is probably normal for someone eating the standard American diet, but societies that eat a mostly or completely vegetarian diet have three regular bowel movements a day. A healthy bowel movement is soft and unformed, not hard or watery and it should breakup when the toilet is flushed. It may have some texture but it shouldn't have much if the food was chewed correctly to begin with. In Ayurveda (the ancient Indian lifestyle science) it is said that "if your stool is sinking, you're sinking" in other words, a proper bowel movement should also float in water. Bowel movements should happen effortlessly, and without straining. If bowel movements have to be forced, if they are painful, or happen less than two or three times a day, the colon is constipated. When the bowel is severally constipated it may produce diarrhea in order to "flush out" hardened fecal with a lot of liquid. Unless diarrhea has become severe and the person is dehydrated, diarrhea should not be stopped, especially with pharmaceutical drugs.

If the average American has only three bowel movements a week and is supposed to have three a day, then by the end of the week they are eighteen bowel movements short. By the end of the month they are seventy-two bowel movements behind. And by the end of a year they have an eight hundred and sixty-four bowel movement deficit. This adds up over the years. When the average person is eighty years old they are about seventy thousand bowel movements behind. No wonder the body starts breaking down and feeling old.

With an understanding of our digestion and elimination, we can focus on correcting our physical weaknesses by learning how to cleanse out old fecal matter that has been accumulating and gluing itself to the bowels over the years.

"I saw few die of hunger- of eating, a hundred thousand."
—Benjamin Franklin

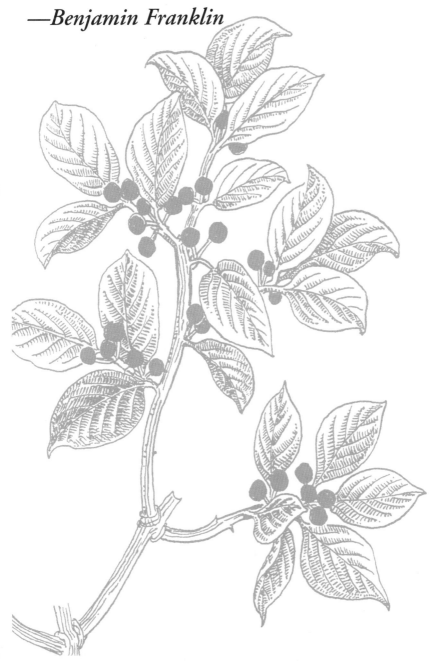

Chapter 2
The Causes of Intestinal Disease

Diet is the leading cause of intestinal disorders. Mucus forming foods cause the bowel to become sluggish and create an ideal environment for bacteria and parasites to thrive. The standard American Diet (SAD), is directly and indirectly responsible for almost every common disease known to medicine.

As staff physician at the Battle Creek Sanitarium for over sixty years, Dr. John Harvey Kellogg witnessed a lot of digestive diseases during his practice. The following few pages are taken form his book, *Colon Hygiene* which he wrote about the causes of intestinal disease:

> **"The use of tobacco.** Numerous laboratory experiments have shown that the use of tobacco in any form has a paralyzing effect upon the splanchnic nerves. Without the aid of these sympathetic nerves normal, rhythmical bowel movements are impossible. The fact that some persons observe an apparently favorable influence from smoking is accepted as evidence that the effects of the weed are favorable to the bowels. These cases are exceptional and misguided. In general, the use of tobacco is highly injurious to the intestine.
>
> **Constipating foods.** There are certain foods and other agents that produce a decided slowing influence upon intestinal movements, either directly or indirectly, through the suppression of the normal stimuli. Liquid foods, such as soups, gruels, porridges, and purees contain so little solid matter that the bulk, considerable though it may be when the food is eaten, is soon reduced to a very small volume. On this account, liquid

foods are almost always constipating. The only exceptions are those liquid foods which contain much sugar, acids or fats.

Pasty cereals such as oatmeal are decidedly constipating in their influence because of their pasty consistency and the little mastication which they generally receive. New bread, hot biscuits, noodles, and doughy foods of all sorts are likewise objectionable.

Fruit juices of all sorts are most suitable for almost all forms of sickness. They contain choice nutrients in a form needing no digestion, ready for immediate absorption and assimilation.

Orange juice or freshly pressed juice of apples, grape, or other sweet or sub-acid fruit, is ideal nourishment for the sick. In the absence of these fresh fruits, dried fruit soaked long in distilled water may furnish a very fair substitute.

Putrefaction. The carmine capsule test shows that in most cases in which the bowels move once daily, the waste disposal function is always several days in arrears. The colon contains the waste and residues of several meals—anywhere from five to twenty or even more—so that there is ample opportunity for the putrefactive process to get well under way.

Putrefaction is the source of the foul odor and gases which originate in the colon, and which are not only most offensive to the sense of smell, but as is well known, are also highly poisonous, and may give rise to nausea, biliousness, loss of appetite, bad breath, dingy skin, headache, Bright's disease, and a host of other grave disorders.

Hasty eating. Insufficient mastication is a fault peculiar to 'civilized' men. The 'savage,' as well as the monkey and all lower animals that are provided with

23

teeth for grinding food, masticates his food with the greatest thoroughness. A skull in the writer's possession shows the teeth of an ancient mound builder, a Malkelkos Indian. The well-worn appearance of the teeth affords sufficient evidence of the thoroughness with which they were used to grind the nuts and cereal foods eaten by ancient Indians.

Meat eating. Carnivorous animals have a short alimentary canal and a smooth colon. The movement of foodstuffs along this short, smooth passage is rapid. This is necessary for the preservation of the life of the animal, as undigested remnants of meat long retained in the body necessarily undergo putrefactive changes with the production of ptomaines and poisons. The digestion of meat leaves much residue, hence a person who lives chiefly on meat suffers from constipation, a condition which favors the putrefaction of undigested food remnants, and this, by creating an alkaline condition of the intestines, paralyzes the bowel and further increases the constipation.

Meat also causes constipation through the fact that it encourages putrefaction of the colon both by introducing harmful organisms in great numbers and by providing material which is best calculated to encourage the growth of these organisms in the colon. Through the putrefaction of undigested remnants of the meat eaten, ammonia and other substances are formed which paralyze the bowel.

The infection of the bowel which results from meat-eating also gives rise to colitis and causes a spastic or contracted condition of the descending colon, a condition found in the most obstinate forms of constipation.

Insufficient fluid. Most persons who suffer from constipation habitually drink too little water. It is difficult to account for this scanty use of a necessity of life, which costs little and is of such inestimable value to the body. Water is far more immediately necessary for the support of life than is food. A man may live six to eight weeks without tasting food in any form, but ten days at the most is the limit of human life without water. The consequence of a scanty use of water is abnormal dryness of the feces, which delays their passage through the lower colon, and often causes an actual stoppage in the pelvic colon or the rectum.

Persons who sweat much, either as the result of hot weather, vigorous exercise, or hot baths, are likely to suffer from constipation, unless special care is taken to supply the body with water sufficient to make good the loss. The skin ordinarily throws off as perspiration an ounce and a half of water each hour, or more than a quart in twenty-four hours. By active exercise or sweating baths, this amount may be increased to thirty or forty ounces in an hour. The kidneys excrete two to three pints daily. It is evident, therefore, that care must be exercised to replace the water that is lost through the skin and the kidneys.

In diabetes, there is a great loss of water through the kidneys. This, also, must be made up by drinking wholesome liquids. If these losses are not made good, the thirsty tissues will absorb as much water as possible from the feces, thus causing hardening and retention in the lower bowel.

Scanty and highly colored urine is an evidence that the tissues are in need of water. Dryness of the skin often testifies to the same need. Water should be taken in proper quantity irrespective of thirst. It may be made palatable by the addition of fresh fruit juices, especially fresh lemon juice.

For the average person a good plan is to take a couple of glasses of water on rising, and the same amount before retiring at night. A glassful should be taken half an hour before dinner and supper, and an equal amount two hours after eating. The free use of oranges or orange juice, and of other juicy fruits, serves the same purpose as water drinking, to the extent of the liquid which they supply.

In all cases in which there is a tendency to dryness of the stools, water should be taken in increased quantity. It is important in such cases, to also diminish the amount of salt eaten. The addition of salt to the food creates thirst for water to dissolve it and to aid in its elimination through the skin and the kidneys.

Children, as well as adults, need much more water than they are usually given. Meat eaters and those who use salt freely require a much larger amount of water than do those who adhere to a low protein diet and who use little salt.

Alcohol and other narcotic drugs. Alcoholic beverages of all sorts tend to produce constipation by causing chronic intestinal catarrh, ulcers of the stomach, and paralysis of the sympathetic nerves.

Resisting the Call The practice of resisting the 'call' of Nature to discharge from the body its accumulated wastes and rubbish is almost universal among 'civilized' people, as the result of a social refinement of manners and modesty which lead to the concealment of certain 'animalistic' body functions. It is important, however, that every person, children as well as adults, should at a very early age be fully instructed respecting the evil results or resisting Nature's call and thus thwarting one of the most important functions of the body.

Colon disease. It is probable that more disease, premature old age death, misery and even crime originate from constipation than from any other bodily disorder.

Constipation is not of itself a disease but a symptom, the cause of which may be disease or simply neglect.

There are several very prevalent errors respecting the colon and its functions which are probably responsible for most of the mischief which arises from disorders of this part of the body.

One of the most universal and damaging errors about the colon is that we conceal its function because of modesty even at the expense of great suffering. Although recent times have given us a greater abundance of restroom facilities, many public places such as grocery stores, malls and shopping plazas, banks and etc., still do not offer adequate facilities either for patrons or passersby. And many of these establishments do not allow use of the restrooms to non-patrons. Such conditions help promote the standard norm of 'holding it,' which is the beginning of bowel dysfunction.

Another modern problem is that in today's fast paced society it has become an inconvenience to take time out to allow the body to cleanse itself and then continue on. There are even accounts from natural healers who have worked with people who had a bowel movement once a month, and even once every other month! This was because of the modern working lifestyles that could not allow a few minutes each day to go to the restroom.

Unfortunately, as we have become more 'civilized,' we have begun to put industry before regularity. Most jobs, and many public schools, do not offer access to restrooms when needed, and the employee or student must postpone their body's desired function to suit the demand of business or convenience. The consequences are most disastrous. The majority of chronic human ills are the results of this neglect.

Another common error which is held by most medical men, as well as by the laity, is that the stool should be 'formed.' This is a false notion that has grown out of the constipation habit which prevails among 'civilized' folk.

The vegetarian Hindus of Armistar, who live chiefly on ground wheat and vegetables, according to Dr. A. H. Browne, have "large, bulky, and not formed, but pultaceous" stools.

A well-formed stool always means constipation. The significance is that the colon is packed full like a sausage and that the fecal matters have been so long retained that they have been compacted by the absorption of water. The whole colon is filled, and the bowel movement is the result of the pressure of the incoming food residues at the other end. When the body's wastes are promptly discharged as they should be, the colon never contains the residues of more than two meals and at the after-breakfast movement should be completely emptied so that the disinfecting and lubricating mucus which its walls secrete may have its opportunity to cleanse and disinfect the body's garbage receptacle, and thus keep it in a sanitary condition.

The California doctor who advised his patient to restrain his desire for a bowel movement at night and hold it until the next morning so that he might have a "well-formed stool," had not the first conception of the normal function of the colon.

The idea that one bowel movement a day is normal and efficient evacuation of the bowels is another error which is universally entertained. One bowel movement a day is a positive indication of constipation. X-ray examinations of the colon after a test meal show that, in persons whose bowels move once a day, the body wastes are usually retained for fifty hours or more. Hurst, of London, and many other authorities finding this condition to be almost universal have been led to regard it as normal, but in this, they are certainly in error. X-ray examinations show that in eight hours from the beginning of a meal the process of digestion has been completed, the digested food has been absorbed, and the unusable residue has been pushed halfway through the colon, and is within two and a half feet of the lower opening of the colon. In eight hours the food has travelled more than twenty-five feet, or ten times the distance which remains to be travelled. The work of digestion is finished, the useful part of the food has been absorbed, there remains nothing to be done but to dispose of the indigestible and useless residue by pushing it along two or three feet further. Certainly no good reason can be assigned for the further retention of the waste matters. It is indeed highly absurd to suppose that forty hours are needed to transport the feces two and a half feet when they have already travelled twenty-five feet in eight hours.

The bowels should move at least three times a day or after each meal. Four movements daily is a still better rhythm and is easily established by a natural regimen, as this the writer has proven in many exceptional cases involving thousands of patients who have been willing to take the time to train their bowels by the means of a proper diet and other simple and natural means."

"If we could give every individual the right amount of nourishment and exercise, not too little and not too much, we would have found the safest way to health."
—*Hippocrates*

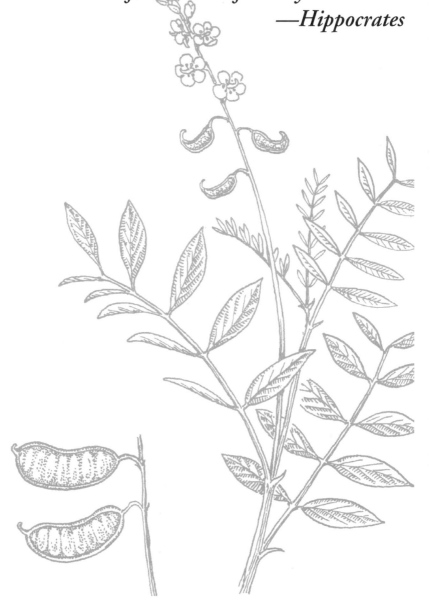

Chapter 3
Healing the Digestive System with Herbs and Natural Therapies

What is the source of intestinal complaints? When we eat unwholesome food, a certain amount of its mucus forming substance stays in the intestine by adhering to the walls. This mucus glues itself on like wallpaper paste and forms layers on the intestinal walls. As each additional layer forms through incorrect eating habits, the muscular and absorptive tissues become thickly covered and proportionately less functional. As these fecal layerings become hardened and continue to grow thicker, eventually only a small opening will remain in the center of the bowel.

We often say, "I have bowel movements every day." Sure, we have bowel movements every day, but what really happens is that our old fecal matter is encrusted on our intestinal walls and prevents the food from being assimilated. Instead of assimilating the nutrition from undigested food, we utilize only ten percent of its real value, and the rest is wasted down the eliminative drain. With the intestinal tract so badly layered and clogged, your food simply cannot get through to the absorptive villi and functional tissues of the intestine. The result is a weakened bowel that loses its elasticity and balloons out.

These hardened layerings in the bowels are just like rings in a tree, which multiply during each year and vary according to the habits and types of materials consumed. When a person suffers from halitosis or bad breath, it's nature's way of saying, "You have a toxic bowel condition."

One patient asked, "Why is it that I only eat one-fifth of what I used to eat, and when I was eating five times as much I had a bowel movement every day, and I thought that was adequate. But now that I am eating only one-fifth of what I

31

formerly ate, I am having from five to seven bowel movements each and every day—and they are massive ones, and I am eating less!!! You figure that one out, will you?"

Well, when I was a boy and working in a cabinet shop, we had an old glue pot. The inside of the pot, as the years rolled on, got smaller and smaller due to the glue adhering to the inside. Because it was a very expensive glue pot, we could not use the hammer on it to break the substance loose, so we had to reverse the process—we had to soak it out! The same is true with the human colon. We have to soak out the old fecal matter to strengthen our colon.

The abnormal intestinal condition that is found among most people today is from improper eating habits that accumulate waste upon the intestinal walls. This waste becomes dehydrated and compacted like dried fruit, or dried flax, and it starts to swell when water gets into it, creating a ballooned pocket in our intestinal tract. A mucus condition in the colon is generally caused by food that gets caught and rots in these pockets, which enemas cannot touch.

Ridding the body of poison is very important, and animal products are the *most* mucus-forming foods. We have thirty-two feet of intestinal tract, and when we plug it up with meat, cheese, milk, etc., the waste materials remain too long and uric acid passes through and toxifies our whole system.

What happens when congestion occurs in the intestines while you are on the Cleansing Program? In one day, with the help of the Lower Bowel herbs, you may soak loose what has been accumulating there during at least a three week layering period of some previous time. The closer the cleansing process approaches the intestinal walls, the harder the encrusted fecal matter is. It is often broken off and comes out in pieces just like an old plastic or rubber hose! A frequent swelling in the abdomen results during the cleanse as the Lower Bowel agents begin soaking through. However, when this filth is cleaned out, you will feel like a million dollars, revitalized and young again.

For instance, in one case we had a boy who for eight months was having somewhat regular and normal bowel movements, then one evening he called his father in the night and was amazed that he had dropped a five pound load, he completely filled the toilet! What had happened was that accumulations from years back had finally broken loose. When this cleansing process is completed, the food value finally returns to the outside intestinal wall, the tissues are fed properly and the peristaltic muscles once again start working.

Now this is why the Lower Bowel Formula is so beneficial, because it is not a crutch. It cleans the liver, the gall bladder, starts the bowel flowing, and stimulates the peristaltic muscles to begin working and kneading out waste. You can take colonics, irrigations, enemas, or herbal laxatives until they are running out your ears, but as long as the peristaltic muscles are not functioning, no permanent healing can be accomplished. So remember, as long as you have a polluted and congested bowel, you are getting only about ten percent of your food value, and your body degenerates as long as this persists.

What are the benefits of a cleansed and properly functioning bowel? The patient mentioned previously who is eating only one-fifth of his former quantity of food now has more strength, more endurance, more pep and energy than he ever had—and he is happier! But these are not the only advantages, especially for those planning to survive the troubled days ahead; for when you become more efficient with your food assimilation within the body, then you will be able to go three to four times as long on the same quantity of food as the average individual. Thus, you will not need as much food to survive during critical times, a regular two year food supply is going to last you eight or nine years. As you clean out and tone up the bowel, you will be assured a greater nutritional efficiency and that all glands and organs will be properly fed and regenerated! When your body is cleansed, you will also be able to assimilate various types of foods and get the food value out of them that nobody else can. Men and women repeatedly raise their hands in our herb classes and volunteer such testi-

33

monials, as "Since we have been on this Cleansing Program, we have cut our food bill straight in half!"

Aids To Heal the Bowel

Suppose you have a case of diarrhea—the majority of people want a remedy that will stop it right away. Diarrhea is simply a condition in which the intestinal tract has become badly clogged and all the fecal solids are being held back allowing only the eliminative liquids to get through. Would you believe it possible for people to have filth in their intestines for five, ten or even more years? We have seen examples of this with our own eyes.

The impurities accumulate with improper diet and lifestyle. When our bodies make an increased effort to clean that wastage out, the dirty channel, or intestinal tract, holds back large materials similar to the way overgrowth and trash can dam an irrigation ditch. When this happens, *do not* try to stop diarrhea, for it is simply the elimination of waste material, but use the appropriate means to remove the obstructing matter and clean the bowel out. The only exception to this rule should be when a person is too weak and the diarrhea is too heavy, in these cases the diarrhea should be stopped with agents such as red raspberry leaves, fresh peaches, dried sunflower leaf tea, etc., then give a mild laxative, followed by other agents that will gently remove the obstruction and build up the area again.

You will be surprised at how much filth three quarts of a stimulating injection will expel. However, injections or enemas are really not the permanent solution for this problem, as they only relieve the condition temporarily, and the peristaltic muscles do not work when enemas are being used for eliminative purposes. Enemas are only a crutch in solving constipation. What is needed here is the Lower Bowel Formula, which is a *corrective food* for the intestinal tract.

In bowel movements, no two people are alike. Often we start the Lower Bowel Formula one capsule three times daily, then reduce to a single capsule a day. When the tonic gets to the outside walls of the intestine and breaks loose some of this hard fecal matter, the old matter will go down the intestines and begin to clog up the tract.

So during your cleansing cycles—when the body is throwing off more of its accumulated wastage, or when the Lower Bowel Formula is getting to the outside of the intestinal tract and breaking loose some of the hard fecal matter from the walls—remember to accentuate or intensify your use of the Lower Bowel Formula and take the necessary quantity to break it loose. When this is accomplished, reduce your dosage.

If you discover undigested food in the fecal matter, this generally means that the bowel is badly clogged so that food is going through the tract without proper assimilation. In addition, when bloating of the bowels occurs, this is a signal that more cleansing is needed. A condition of sciatic rheumatism will always develop where the sigmoid portion of the lower bowel becomes congested, and the toxic poisons from the bowel are subsequently absorbed by the adjacent area, irritating the nerves controlling the sacroiliac and, in turn, throwing it out of place—and so goes the vicious cycle!

A periodic purification and cleansing of the lower intestinal tract is very important for us. This is your sewage system—and when the eliminative function is efficient and clean, you do not have to worry about sluggishness or toxification in the body.

On the next few pages is a list of herbs and natural therapies in alphabetical order. Each therapy may be used by itself or as part of a complete program for healing the digestive system.

Therapies

Abdominal Massage

    Many times intestinal blockages can be "massaged out" using a simple technique. Using both hands, gently massage the abdomen, starting from the sufferers's lower right side near the hip bone and slowly up to the rib cage. Continue across under the rib cage and then massage downwards in a straight line to the other hip bone. Massage across from the left hip bone to the right and then start again. Use light to moderate pressure making sure the massage does not cause pain to increase.

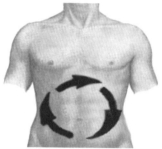

    This massage will often relieve stubborn intestinal blockages that do not respond well to other treatments. Abdominal massage can be performed several times a day. Be careful not to massage too deeply, several organs are close to the surface of the abdomen and could be damaged by too much pressure.

Apple Cider Vinegar and Honey

    Apple cider is both oxygenating and alkalinizing to the gastrointestinal system. It helps stimulate digestive enzyme production in the stomach and intestine as well alkalinize the rest of the body. Many have used the combination of apple cider and honey to lose weight, alleviate arthritis, desolve bone spurs, and rid themselves of kidney and gall stones. Mix one tablespoon of apple cider and one tablespoon of honey in a glass of distilled water. Do this three times daily. For the best results use organic, raw, and unfiltered apple cider and honey.

Cabbage and Carrot Juice

Cabbage has been a old fashion remedy for ulcerative conditions for hundreds of years. This use has been substantiated by scientific studies [1]. N.W. Walker states in his book *Fresh Vegetable and Fruit Juices* that "Duodenal ulcers have responded almost miraculously to the drinking of cabbage juice. The only drawback is the frequent generation of excessive gas. In this case, plain carrot juice has been used with equal success and most people find it more palatable."

Castor Oil Fomentations (*Ricinus communis*)

This thick oil, cold pressed from the seeds of the castor plant is a strong purgative and should not be used internally unless directed by a health care professional with experience with this substance. Externally it can be very cleansing and drawing. Fomentations of the oil are used by herbalists to cleanse congested and painful organs such as the liver, spleen, gallbladder, pancreas, and bowel. Many have reported a small amount of castor oil in the stool after a castor oil fomentation, this is a sign that the oil is being absorbed into the body.

Castor Oil Fomentation Procedure:

1. Soak a flannel or natural cotton cloth in castor oil. Wring it out slightly so it does not drip.
2. Apply the soaked cloth to the skin over the affected organ. Place some plastic over the castor oil soaked cloth to protect clothing and bedding from the oil.
3. Place a hot towel over the cloth and plastic layer, and then a hot water bottle or heating pad on top of the hot towel. It is recommended that you also apply cold packs to the fomentation (twelve minutes hot and four minutes cold). This method takes more effort but is more effective than just the heat when dealing with pain and congestion.
4. The fomentation should be kept warm (unless both hot and cold are used) from thirty minutes to one hour.
5. Wash the area with warm water and natural soap if

needed.

6. Repeat three to four times a day for six days or until the condition is cleared.

Catnip and Fennel
Catnip (*Nepeta cataria*)
Fennel (*Foeniculum vulgare*)

This herbal combination has been used for hundreds of years to ease stomach problems including colic, stomachache, and stomach cramps. It can be found in Dr. Christopher's Catnip and Fennel tincture or in the Kid-e-Col combination for children. It can also be made as a tea at home.

Cayenne (*Capsicum spp.*)

Cayenne is a wonderful remedy for bleeding ulcers[2]. It stops bleeding and starts healing the mucus membrane of the stomach and intestinal tract. It is recommended that you start with only 1/8 teaspoon three times a day, and then gradually work up to one full teaspoon three times a day

A lady who had been attending Dr. Christopher's lectures over the years told the story of her husband who had a severe case of stomach ulcers. The doctor recommended that part of the stomach be removed, but the man preferred to suffer the pain rather than risk such an operation. But he also ridiculed his wife's recommendations to use Cayenne and other herbs. Whenever he would see Dr. Christopher in town, he'd bellow, "Hello, Doc! Killed anybody with Cayenne today?" Naturally, Dr. Christopher tried to avoid him, but one day he came directly to the Doctor—but this time without any sarcasm, instead being very apologetic, telling this story.

He had come home from work one night, so sick he wanted to die, with stomach ulcers. His wife was not home, but he was in such pain that he decided to commit suicide. When he looked into the medicine cabinet to find some kind of medicine poisonous enough to kill him, he discovered that his wife had discarded all the old bottles of pharmaceutical medicines. All he could find were some bottles of herbs and a large container of Cayenne pepper. He figured that a large dose of that would kill him, so he took a heaping tablespoon in a glass of hot water, gulped it down, rushed into the bedroom, and covered his head with a pillow so that the neighbors couldn't hear his dying screams.

The next thing he knew, his wife was shaking him awake the next morning. He had slept all night, the first time in years, instead of waking every half hour or so for antiacid tablets. To his amazement, all his pain was gone. He continued using the Cayenne faithfully, three times a day, and never had any more trouble with ulcers.

Colonics

A colonic is the introduction of a large amount of liquid into the colon using gravity for an internal bath that helps cleanse the colon of toxins, gas, and accumulated fecal matter. Unlike an enema, it does not involve the retention of water. During a proper colonic treatment there should be little discomfort, and almost no internal pressure, just a steady gentle flow of warm water in and out of the colon. At the same time, an abdominal massage (as described on page 36) can help stimulate the colon to eliminate old deposits.

Colonics can be an effective part of internal cleansing if performed correctly. They should not be relied upon as the sole means of cleansing the bowel because they do not rebuild or nourish the tissue. Colonics are sometimes necessary in cases of severe toxicity and constipation but may become habit forming if used too regularly. Usually only a few colonics are all that is needed before relying solely on herbal formulas and a good diet to cleanse and nourish the bowel.

Confectionery Type Bowel Aid

Make these delicious candies using the following instructions as a basic guide and vary as you wish. To each pint of chopped or ground up dried fruit (raisins, prunes, apricots, peaches, apples, dates, figs, etc.), mix in one ounce powdered flaxseed, one ounce powdered licorice root, one ounce powdered slippery elm bark, and add enough sorghum or blackstrap molasses to mold it into small balls. Roll these in equal parts, powdered carob and slippery elm bark so the confection is not sticky. Use these as needed. The ingredients and amounts can be adjusted to taste.

Enemas

An enema involves the injection of a solution into the rectum and lower bowel to soften the feces, and cleanse the colon. Enemas may be used occasionally to relieve constipation and deliver herbal medicines to the lower bowel. If used too often, enemas become habit forming and the body relies on their action to have a normal bowel movement.

A regular adult enema consists of one to two quarts of liquid, enemas for children or those with a weak or constipated bowel should be less (as low as a half a cup). A variety of liquids may be used for different purposes such as catnip tea, for calming the stomach and bowel and relieving cramping; distilled water and wheat grass juice for alkalinizing the body; or distilled water by itself for general cleansing and hydrating the bowel. The temperature of the enema should be slightly below body temperature (98.6 F). This aids the body in retaining the enema for a greater amount of time.

During the administration of an enema, the recipient lies on their left side, with the right leg flexed. This position will enable the enema solution to flow easily into the rectum and colon. A slant board may also be used to allow the enema to reach the transverse and the descending colon. After an enema is administered, massage the abdomen as described earlier. The enema should be retained until the massage is complete (less than five minutes). Sometimes it is necessary to repeat this procedure until the liquid exiting the rectum is mostly clear. Take care when inserting the enema tube into the rectum. The lining of the rectum and colon can be punctured by the plastic tube if it is forced in.

Exercise

To maintain good intestinal health, it is good practice to exercise. In all forms of exercise one should remember that the body areas firm up and strengthen themselves with exercise up to, that is until, the time of fatigue. Continuing on after fatigue, exercise loses value rapidly. Just before the time of tiring, stop and rest before continuing on. Gradually, exercising will become easier and stamina will increase without fatigue or damage. One of the best and most enjoyable types of exercise is to walk with a long stride from the hips, increasing each day the length of time doing it. Swimming, dancing, and jogging are all beneficial if not overdone.

The following is an excerpt taken from *Colon Hygiene* by Dr. John Harvey Kellogg, M.D. Here, he gives a good explanation of what exercises are useful when dealing with intestinal problems.

"**Exercise.** Bodily activity is another way of mechanically stimulating the intestine. Vigorous exercise sets the diaphragm and abdominal muscles at work in such a way that the intestines are, between the two, vigorously kneaded and squeezed and thus stimulated into action.

Every farmer knows the constipating effect of idleness upon his horses and cattle. Most observing persons have noted in their own experience the advantage of taking a brisk walk before or after breakfast.

The sedentary man or woman not only loses the immediate effect which results from the increased activity of the diaphragm and abdominal muscles, but his abdominal muscles become permanently weakened, relaxed, lacking in tone, and incapable of supporting the intestines in their proper place, thus adding a number of other factors which contribute very materially to the lessening of intestinal activity.

The excellent effects that walking has upon

bowel activity are well known. Riding is also of great advantage in the same way. These exercises, and many others, mechanically stimulate the colon as well as all parts of the intestinal tract by communicating to it a continued series of slight shocks, by which reflex movements are excited. The active play of children is as necessary to maintain proper bowel action as for muscular development. The movements of skipping, hopping and jumping are especially useful because they induce sudden vigorous contractions of the abdominal muscles and vigorous diaphragm movements by which the colon is compressed and stimulated. The folk dancing of the Middle Ages, which has been revived in recent years, is to be highly commended as a health measure for the above reasons.

Those whose occupations are such as to give them plenty of exercise are fortunate in being able to lead lives which in large measure conform to natural requirements. Such persons never need suffer from constipation if they eat proper food, drink an abundance of water—at least three to five pints daily—and take care to give the bowels an opportunity for movement after each meal, and a prompt evacuation whenever there is a 'call.'

Those who are compelled to lead sedentary lives must take daily and regular exercise of a sort calculated to benefit the bowels if they would escape the evils of constipation and its sedentary results.

Exercises which combat constipation. The exercises that are of the greatest value in cases of constipation are those which bring into strong action the muscles of the abdomen. The abdominal muscles are generally weak and relaxed, and the intra-abdominal pressure is consequently low.

By appropriate exercises the weak muscles may be strengthened, the intra-abdominal pressure may be raised and the colon may be thus enabled to contract with sufficient impetus to expel its contents.

Hill climbing, Hill climbing is a more valuable exercise than walking on level ground because the abdominal muscles are brought into more active play. When mountain climbing is not an available form of exercise, nearly the same results may be obtained by climbing a ladder or by walking up and down stairs. The writer has also made use of the treadmill as the means of securing muscular exercise similar to that required in hill climbing.

Horseback riding, Horseback riding is especially indicated as an exercise for constipation. However, persons accustomed to riding must ride a considerable distance or ride a hard trotting horse for this to be an effective exercise.

Rowing, is one of the very best exercises to combat constipation, provided the chest is held high during the exercise, and especially if care is taken to give the trunk as strong a backward movement as possible. But one must avoid holding the trunk forward with the shoulders rounded and the chest depressed.

Tennis, is highly recommended for young persons and those who are sufficiently strong to engage in this form of exercise without injury. This very popular game is, however, too vigorous for persons with weak hearts.

The Medicine Ball, This is a capital exercise for persons who are sufficiently strong. It brings the muscles of the trunk into vigorous action.

Work exercises, The movements of chopping, digging, swinging the hammer and mowing are highly valuable exercises if taken with due care to maintain the body in an erect position. Many household occupations, such as scrubbing, washing, and general housework are excellent forms of exercise when the correct posture is maintained."

Fruits and Vegetables (Raw)

Use plenty of fresh, ripe fruit, or un-sulphured dried fruit, lots of raw fibrous vegetables to chew on, or use in salads, and small amounts of whole bran—the type supplied by the millers or from a health store. Add honey and water, or fresh fruit or vegetable juice to moisten the bran for easier eating. The person using plenty of whole uncracked low-heated grains does not need additional bran as a rule.

The test for wholesome live grains is that after presoaking and low-heating (under 140 F), they are still alive and will grow. If you have some individual whole grain (wheat, buckwheat, rye, millet, barley, flaxseed) single or in your favorite combination left over after a meal, and/or some whole grain as a base used for a casserole, take some of these grains out and plant them in a row or furrow in the backyard. In another row, plant some wheat flakes, granola and a loaf of bread, cover them, water and care for this new little garden and see which row will sprout and grow. The row that produces is the wholesome (Webster's unabridged dictionary defines wholesome as "with the life therein as in its original state") food that is alive and will give life to your body. The row that remains dormant is dead and is only a filler without true life in it.

Garlic Implant (*Allium sativum*)

Garlic has been used for centuries as both an antibacterial and antiparasitic. It has shown its effectiveness as a antibiotic in clinical trials many times[3]. In cases of intestinal parasites and infection of the colon it is sometimes necessary to use a garlic implant. For this treatment, blend three average sized cloves of garlic in two cups water. This implant is then placed in the lower bowel either with a bulb syringe or enema. This should be retained for ten to fifteen minutes while the abdomen is massaged.

Ginger (*Zingiber officinale*)

Ginger has been shown to have cholesterol lowering, anti-inflammatory and anti-nausea properties in clinical studies[4]. One of the principle uses of ginger has been for morning sickness. Morning sickness effects between 70%-85% of all pregnant women and ginger has been shown to lessen the severity and the duration of these incidents[5]. Other uses include colitis, nausea, irritable bowel syndrome, and seasickness. Ginger comes in many forms, candied, powdered, syrup, tea, and tablets. Ginger is a lower body tonic, and has been used to treat intestinal and reproductive problems. Ginger root has been used as a medicine for thousands of years and has been shown to be both safe and effective.

Herbal Gruel

Flax or psyllium (*Linum usitatissimum* or *Plantago ovata*)
Licorice (*Glycyrrhiza glabra*)
Marshmallow (*Althea officinals*)
Comfrey (*Symphytum officinale*)
Lobelia (*Lobelia inflata*)

If you desire additional assistance to the bowel, prepare flaxseed and/or psyllium seed, licorice root, marshmallow root, and comfrey root, each in three parts, and add one part lobelia herb. Sweeten with honey if desired. Use as little or as much as you require for assisting in free, easy bowel movements. The flaxseed and the psyllium seed give bulk; licorice root is a mild aperient (mildest of laxatives); marshmallow root is used to assist clearance where hard stools are prevalent; comfrey root is the healer and rebuilder of weak areas and gives lubrication; and lobelia is the accentuating herb.

Immucalm

Astragalus (*Astragalus membranaceus*)
Marshmallow (*Althea officinalis*)
    This combination is used to strengthen the immune system while making it less "hypersensitive." It is often used in cases of allergy or autoimmune disorders such as arthritis, Type I Diabetes, Multiple Sclerosis, and Crohn's Disease. The standard dosage is two capsules three times daily. Many people find that higher amounts are sometimes needed when first taking this formula. Many herbalists recommend starting with five capsules three times daily for the first week or two and then continuing with the standard dose until desired results are achieved.

Intestinal Sweeper (Dr. Christopher's)

    To assist in keeping the bowels clean, and feeding and nourishing them at the same time, add a fouth a cup or more flaxseed and/or psyllium seed to the whole, uncracked grains being prepared for breakfast or noonday meal as is explained on the low heating procedure in *Dr. Christopher's Three Day Cleanse and Mucusless Diet* and the *Transfiguration Diet*

Juices and Water

    An abundant supply of wholesome unsweetened fruit and vegetable juice (especially raw spinach juice) should be used daily. In addition, drink plenty of distilled water to supply liquid to the body. The human body under normal circumstances is made up of between seventy five and eighty percent fluid; this must be replenished daily in the form of liquid intake. Only the best of liquid should be used to replace the daily loss through elimination from urination, perspiration and from the bowel area, etc. The use of inorganic drinks and beverages high in sugar, synthetic sweetenings, chemical additives and artificial colorings (soft drinks), the use of alcoholic beverages and polluted stream or tap waters is as ridiculous as pouring salt, sugar or dirty water into the gas tank of your car.

In his book *Fresh Vegetable and Fruit Juices*, Norman W. Walker, D.Sc., wrote about the benefits of juicing and how it affects health.

"When the food is raw, whether whole or in the form of juice, every atom in such food is vital and organic. Therefore, the oxalic acid in our raw vegetables and their juices is organic, and is not only beneficial, but essential for physiological functions of the body.

The oxalic acid in cooked and processed foods, however, is definitely dead, or inorganic, and as such is positively both pernicious and destructive. Oxalic acid readily combines with calcium. If these are both organic, the result is a beneficial constructive combination, as the former helps the digestive assimilation of the latter, at the same time stimulating the peristaltic functions of the body.

When the oxalic acid becomes inorganic by cooking or processing the foods that contain it, then this acid forms an interlocking compound with the calcium, even combining with the calcium in other foods eaten during the same meal, destroying the nourishing value of both. This results in such a serious deficiency of calcium that it has even been known to cause decomposition of the bones (osteoporosis). This is the reason I never eat cooked or canned spinach.

As to the oxalic acid itself, when converted into an inorganic acid by cooking or processing the food, it often results in causing inorganic oxalic acid crystals to form in the kidneys.

It is worthy of notice that the minerals in our foods, iron, for example, frequently cannot be assimilated and used completely if they have become inorganic through cooking, and often prevent the utilizing of other elements through chemical and other action. Thus, the iron in fresh, raw spinach juice may be utilized 100%, but only one-fifth of that, or less, would be available in cooked spinach.

It is well to bear in mind, therefore, that as the organic oxalic acid is so vital to our well-being, the fresh raw juice of the vegetables containing it should be used daily to supplement the eating of these raw vegetables included in our daily salads. The most abundant supply of organic oxalic acid is found in fresh raw spinach and rhubarb."

Papaya Cleanse

Fresh papaya is high in natural enzymes (mostly papain) which help the body digest food and old deposits in the lower bowel. The papaya cleanse is simple, eat papaya and drink distilled water for two days. Remember to eat some of the pungent papaya seeds (they aid digestion). This cleanse not only jump-starts digestion but can rid the body of some long standing health problems such as allergies, bad breath, and chronic constipation.

Parasite Cleanse

A constipated and toxic bowel is the perfect environment for parasites who live off of dead and decaying matter. Simply changing this environment through cleansing and diet will often eliminate parasites. Sometimes it is also necessary to use an herb or herbal formula to help the body expel or destroy parasites. In these stubborn cases Dr. Christopher's Intestinal Parasite Syrup (VF Syrup) can aid the body in getting rid of these unwanted pests. The recommended dosage is one teaspoonful each morning and night for three days. On the fourth day drink one cup of Senna and Peppermint tea, using a half a teaspoon of each in a cup of hot, distilled water. Rest two days and repeat two more times. Single herbs that are helpful include garlic, pumpkin seeds, wormwood, black walnut bark, and clove powder. Symptoms of parasitic infestation may include one or more of the following: anal itching, diarrhea, abdominal pain, cramping, nausea, weight loss, fatigue, and distended abdomen.

Posture

The following is taken from *Colon Hygiene* by John Harvey Kellogg, M.D.

"**Posture exercises,** Maintenance of an erect position of the trunk is of first importance of persons suffering from constipation. When the chest is lowered, as in sitting in a relaxed attitude, the distance between the breastbone and the pelvis is diminished so that the large muscles which form the front of the abdominal wall are shortened and relaxed. In this attitude, the muscles cannot be contracted sufficiently to produce the proper degree of intra-abdominal pressure. When the chest is held high, the rectus muscles are stretched, and are thus able by contraction to produce the maximum effect in compressing the colon. Flat-chested persons are predisposed to constipation because of inefficient action of the abdominal muscles.

The ordinary chair must be regarded to a very considerable degree as responsible for the prevalence of flat chest and round shoulders, and the evils which result from this deformity. It is possible to sit in an erect attitude in a chair of any shape, but with a chair with a straight back, a constant effort of forcible contraction of the muscles is required to maintain the body in an erect position. The moment the muscles are permitted to relax, the trunk falls into an abnormal and unhealthy attitude, the spinal column being curved backward instead of forward, as is natural and necessary for health.

As the results of an habitually wrong attitude in sitting, the same improper attitude is maintained when standing and walking, and the figure becomes deformed. A flat chest, round shoulders, and a forward carriage of the hips are characteristics to be found in the great majority of persons who lead sedentary lives, especially those who sit much at their work, such as accountants, writers, teachers, and professional people generally. One of the first things, then, for a constipated person to do is to correct his standing and sitting attitudes. This may be done by careful execution of the following exercises, which the writer has employed for more than 25 years with much satisfaction in the treatment of cases of this sort.

Posture, A stooped or relaxed posture when sitting or standing tends strongly to induce constipation by weakening the abdominal muscles and causing congestion of the liver and all other abdominal organs. The viscera, overfilled with blood, and lacking the support of the abdominal muscles, becomes prolapsed. The colon falls with the rest; the intestinal contents stagnate; the bowel becomes distended; the ileocecal valve becomes incompetent; infection travels up the small intestine, and a long list of ills result.

An erect posture secures proper exercise of the muscles of the trunk, correct breathing, normal circulation of blood in the viscera, and promotes in a high degree normal bowel movement.

A further cause of injury is the lowering of the diaphragm and diminished action of this important muscle, which when normally active applies to the colon and other active viscera a sort of rhythmic massage which is a valuable aid to bowel action.

To correct the standing posture. Stand against a straight wall. Place heels, hips, shoulders, head and hands firmly against the wall. Now bend the head backwards as far as possible, or until the eyes look straight up to the ceiling, at the same time permitting the chest and shoulders to move forward. While holding the head in this position, press the hands firmly against the wall. Draw the chin down to position without allowing the shoulders to move backward, still holding the body rigid, allowing the arms to fall at the sides. In this position the chest will be held high and the abdominal muscles well drawn in. While holding this position, execute movements with the arms, raising them above the head in swimming movements, etc.

This is the correct standing position and should, as much as possible, be constantly maintained in standing and walking. It is impossible, of course, to hold the muscles constantly rigid. In relaxing, however, care should be taken to keep the chest forward, so that the body does not fall back into the former incorrect attitude.

Exercises to correct the sitting posture. When sitting upon a chair or stool, preferably the latter, proceed as follows:

Place the hands on the hips with the thumbs behind. Bend the head backwards so as to look straight up at the ceiling, then bend forward as far as possible while still keeping the eyes on the ceiling. Make firm pressure with the thumbs, and while pressing hard, bring the body up to the erect position. Still keeping the eyes upon the ceiling, holding the elbows back as far as possible, and without lessening the pressure of the thumbs, bring the chin down to position.

If this movement is executed according to directions, it will bring the body into perfect position, with the chest raised high and the abdominal muscles well drawn in."

Probiotics

The intestine is host to millions of microorganisms. These organisms are called your intestinal flora. Some of the bacteria living in your intestine help digest food and produce nutrients that are essential to your health such as vitamin K, vitamin B12, and biotin. When the intestinal environment is disturbed, sometimes the intestinal flora becomes out of balance. Symptoms include flatulence, diarrhea, candida infections etc. This can happen with antibiotic use, drug use, chronic diarrhea, and sugar consumption. Probiotics and fermented foods such as rejuvalac, sauerkraut, kimchi (kimchee), and vinegar help restore balance to the intestine.

Psyllium seed and husk (*Plantago ovata, Plantago ispaghula*)
Psyllium comes from the Greek word 'psylla' meaning flea, because the tiny seed resembles a flea. Psyllium husks are pure dietary fiber, composed mostly of cellulose. They are not digested in the small intestine, but are partially broken down in the colon. They act as a broom in the intestinal tract, scraping and cleansing out toxins and deposits. Psyllium seeds and husks swell as they absorb water and waste material in the bowels. This forms a soft, bulky mass that passes through the colon quickly (eliminating potentially toxic waste from the colon). Psyllium seeds or husks have a unique action in the bowels; they can be used to either stop diarrhea or help with constipation. The main difference between seed and husk action is that the seed acts more like a broom to the intestine, scraping away old deposits. The husks form more bulk, making bowel movements more solid and less watery.

Take one teaspoon husk or seed (approximately five grams) stir into a glass of water and drink immediately (before it thickens). Follow this seven minutes later with another glass of water. Psyllium may be taken this way three times per day if needed. Two capsules of psyllium may also be taken but should be immediately followed by two glasses of water. It is often necessary to take psyllium with a laxative combination like Dr. Christopher's Lower Bowel Formula to prevent the psyllium from fermenting in the intestines causing gas and bloating.

Rebounding
Unlike most forms of exercise, rebounding affects every single cell, muscle and organ in the body. The results, when used for even two or three minutes, two or three times a day, can be amazing. Rebounders are not just mini-

trampolines, their springs are tapered. Regular mini-tramps repeatedly strain the knees with jerky motions, the tapered springs of a quality rebounder are designed to protect the knees. At the bottom of each bounce, they slow the decent gradually (absorbing the impact), causing less stress and less injury. Rebounding can increase circulation, increases mobility, stimulate weight loss, improve muscle tone, relieve pain, reduce stress and tension, stimulate metabolism, boost the immune systems, improve eyesight, and stimulate lymphatic circulation.

Reflexology

Reflexive areas in the feet correspond to internal organs throughout the body. These reflex areas can be used to stimulate healing and improve the function of the bowels.

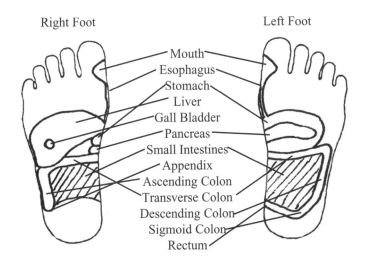

Right Foot   Left Foot

Mouth
Esophagus
Stomach
Liver
Gall Bladder
Pancreas
Small Intestines
Appendix
Ascending Colon
Transverse Colon
Descending Colon
Sigmoid Colon
Rectum

Reflexology Treatment for the Colon

Following the reflex chart above, locate the ascending colon reflex area on the bottom of the right foot. Steady the foot using one hand and gently massage the reflex area upward towards the toes. Continue this movement on the transverse colon reflex massaging from left to right. Next locate the transverse colon reflex of the left foot and massage it from left

53

to right. Massage the descending colon reflex of the left foot with downward movements and then continue across the sigmoid colon toward the rectum reflex. During this reflexology treatment make smooth motions with your thumbs and picture yourself moving toxins out of the body. This treatment should last between five and ten minutes. Water should be given afterwards to aid the body in removing these toxins.

Another reflex to the lower bowel is on the sides of each leg. Simply massage the side of the upper leg from the hip to the knee, moving downwards only. Do this for five to fifteen minutes several times a day. This procedure is most effective in children and infants, but it works in adults and animals as well.

Slant Board Routine

Gravity has a strong effect on the entire body especially the digestive system. The colon has to work against gravity everyday, as it moves food through the small intestine and up and out of the large intestine. In cases of a prolapsed bowel or distended colon it is helpful to reverse gravity's effect. One way to do this is using a slantboard. A slantboard is a simple device made from a long board, one end propped up on a low chair or couch and the other resting on the floor. A slantboard should be wide and long enough to fit your body, as well as strong enough to support your weight. It should be padded enough to be comfortable and so a person can lie down on the board without sliding off.

The herbal combination that we use in the Slant Board Routine is Dr. Christopher's Prolapse Combination. It consists of six parts oak bark (*Quercus alba*), three parts mullein (*Verbascum thapsus*), four parts yellow dock root (*Rumex crispus*), three parts black walnut bark or leaves (*Juglans nigra*), six parts comfrey root (*Symphytum officinale*), one part lobelia (*Lobelia inflata*), and three parts marshmallow root (*Althea officinalis*). A concentrated tea of this herbal formula is used as a rectal injection. To concentrate a tea, add two ounces of herb to two pints of hot water. After the tea has steeped, remove the herbs and simmer until the liquid is reduced to one pint.

Dr. Christopher's Slant Board Routine:

1. Make an enema of concentrated tea.
2. Administer the enema while lying on the slantboard (head downwards). Gravity will draw the tea into the transverse colon and start to heal the bowel.
3. Massage the abdomen for at least five minutes while on the slantboard. After the massage the enema may be eliminated. Then return and lie on the slantboard for another ten minutes.
4. This may be repeated twice a day.

Slant boards are also used to relieve stress and fatigue by taking pressure off the body's organs and allowing them to shift into a more natural placement.

Slippery Elm and Licorice Root Gruel
(Gastro-Intestinal Formula)
Slippery Elm Bark Powder *(Ulmus rubra)*
Licorice Root Powder (*Glycyrrhiza glabra*)
This soothing herbal combination is not commercially available but has helped many people with ulcerative colitis, Crohn's disease, irritable bowel syndrome, ulcers, and other digestive disorders. Mix three parts slippery elm to one part licorice root in cold water. The consistency of the gruel should be similar to thin Cream of Wheat. The standard dosage is a tablespoon full every other waking hour. More may also be taken throughout the day for relief of intestinal pain. This herbal food soothes inflamed tissue and rebuilds areas that have been damaged.

Licorice is a traditional Chinese remedy for stomach as well as respiratory problems. It has a 3000 year history of safe use when it is used in its natural unaltered form. Concentrated extracts of licorice have a higher amount of glycyrrhizinic acid which has been known to cause hypertension, water and sodium retention, and loss of potassium. Licorice in its whole, unconcentrated form has naturally occurring levels of glycyrrhizinic acid and does not cause these symptoms.

Many studies have been performed on the gastrointestinal healing properties of licorice[6]. Research has shown that licorice-derived compounds can raise the concentration of prostaglandins in the digestive system. Prostaglandins promote mucous secretion from the stomach, as well as stimulate the stomach lining to produce new healthy cells. It was also shown that licorice prolongs the life span of stomach cells and has an antipepsin (antacid) effect. This combined medicinal action makes licorice a perfect healer for gastrointestinal diseases.

The hydrophilic mucilage in slippery elm produces a soothing coat in the digestive tract[7]. It tastes slightly sweet and has a light maple fragrance. This herb has been used for centuries to treat gastrointestinal complaints. It coats the alimentary canal and provides nutrients and a soothing, protective environment for the body to repair damage. Slippery elm can also be used on wounds and decubitus ulcers on the outside of the body. The nutritive properties of slippery elm have even made it a perfect first food for infants. Slippery elm is often given to those who have stomach problems and "can't hold anything down". Slippery elm has the tendency to remain in the stomach and intestines and is not regurgitated with other foods.

Super-Lax
Aloe (*Aloe vera*)
Senna Leaves and Pods (*Senna alexandrina*)
Cascara Sagrada Bark (*Rhamnus purshiana*)
Gentian Root (*Gentiana lutea*)
Ginger Rhizome (*Zingiber officinale*)
Garlic (*Allium sativum*)
Cayenne Pepper (*Capsicum spp.*)
Turkey Rhubarb (*Rheum officinales*)

56

Flax seed (*Linum usitatissimum*)

This potent formula stimulates peristaltic action and over time, strengthens the muscles of the large intestine. It halts putrefaction and disinfects, soothes and heals the mucus membrane lining of your entire digestive tract. This herbal tonic improves digestion, increases the flow of bile which in turn cleans the gall bladder, bile ducts and the liver. It is stronger than the Lower Bowel Formula but not as intense as Quick Colon Formula #1.

Kid-E-Reg
Slippery Elm Bark (*Ulmus rubra*)
Licorice Root (*Glycyrrhiza glabra*)
Fennel Seed (*Foeniculum vulgare*)
Anise Seed (*Pempinella anisum*)
Fig Syrup (*Ficus carica*)

This non-laxative liquid formula for children supports the bowel and digestive system. It is both gentle and effective for mild constipation and bowel irritation. This formula is also designed to ease flatulence and upset stomach. The herbs and fruit it contains are sweet and designed to be easy for children to take.

Lobelia (*Lobelia inflata*)

The alkaloids in lobelia stimulate the vagus nerve which controls the stomach. A small amount of lobelia has the effect of calming the stomach, decreasing nausea, and relieving stomach cramps. Larger amounts of lobelia have been known to act as a purgative, emptying the stomach of its contents. Dr. Samuel Thompson stated that "There is no vegetable which the earth produces more harmless in its effect on the human system, and none more powerful in removing disease and promoting health than lobelia." Lobelia works best when used in conjunction with catnip, peppermint, or cayenne. Also, due to its alkaloid content, lobelia extracts made with vinegar are more effective than those made with alcohol and water. Five to ten drops of the tincture are usually sufficient to relieve an upset stomach.

Lower Bowel Formula (Fen-LB or Herbal LB)
Barberry bark (*Berberis vulgaris*)
Cascara sagrada bark (*Rhamnus purshiana*)
Cayenne (*Capsicum spp.*)
Ginger (*Zingiber officinalis*)
Golden Seal root (*Hydrastis canadensis*)
Lobelia herb and/or seeds (*Lobelia inflata*)
Red Raspberry leaves (*Rubus idaeus*)
Turkey rhubarb root (*Rheum palmatum*)
Fennel (*Foeniculum officinale*)

Over a period of time, the mucusless diet, with its fiber from whole grains and from fruits, vegetables, nuts and seeds will regulate bowel function. However, with a buildup of layers of mucus linings as coatings on the bowel walls, it is best to use herbs that are specific in toning, rebuilding and strengthening this area. We do not recommend laxatives such as those purchased from a drug store, or herbal laxatives from health food stores that are *just* laxatives. These become habit forming. Instead, we recommend using herbs to feed and rebuild the bowel, to activate the dormant peristaltic muscles and clean off the bowel walls for complete assimilation of foods going through the intestinal tract. That is why we recommend using Dr. Christopher's Lower Bowel Formula. It is strong enough to work on the most constipated bowel, yet gentle enough to use everyday.

Take according to how many you need. As there are no two people alike in age, size, or physical constitution, and the bowel itself will differ in persons as much as fingerprints, most people will start with two single 'O' capsules three times a day, and then regulate the dosage from there. If the stool seems too loose, then cut down; but if it is difficult to get a bowel movement and the stool is hard and takes a long time to eliminate, then increase the amount until the stools become soft and loosely formed. In very difficult cases, you could take even up to forty of these capsules a day, since these herbs are only *food* and do no damage to you. After the hard material has broken loose and is eliminating more freely, the copious amounts of eliminating matter will gradually decrease (these are hard encrustations of fecal matter that have been stored in the bowel for many years that are breaking loose and soaking up intestinal liquids). But do not reduce the Lower Bowel Formula dosage so much at this point that you lose the advantageous momentum and continuity of elimination. In most cases, the improper diet has caused the peristaltic muscles to quit working, and it will take six to nine months with the aid of the Lower Bowel Formula for the average individual to clean out the old fecal matter and rebuild the bowel structure sufficiently, and have these muscles work entirely on their own.

Most of us have pounds of old, dried fecal matter that is stored up in the colon, is toxifing the system, and keeping the food from being assimilated. Because of this putrefied condition, we engorge ourselves with many times more than the actual body requirements. In the process we wear out our bodies in trying to get sufficient food value and are still always hungry and eating. Whereas after the bowel is cleansed, the food is readily assimilated and the person can sustain himself on about one-third the quantity of his current food consumption with four or five times an increase in power, energy, vitality and life.

The clean body is able to assimilate the simple food values through the cell structures in the colon instead of being trapped in a maze of wastage and inhibited by the hard fecal casing on the intestinal walls where the largest part of the nutritional substance becomes pushed on and eliminated before it can do any good. When the body is completely clean, the Lower Bowel Formula will no longer be necessary—then your food will be your medicine and your medicine will be your food. Once the bowel is cleansed, this Lower Bowel Formula should only be used as needed, providing you have stayed on the program properly. Each ingredient in the Lower Bowel Formula is explained here in detail.

Ingredients of the Lower Bowel Formula:

Barberry *(Berberis vulgaris)*
If this is not available you may substitute Oregon Grape root *(Berberis aquifolium)*, also called Rocky Mountain Grape root, which is the same family and will do the same type of job. This family of herbs acts as a specific for the liver and gall bladder (hepatic) area causing the bile to flow freely instead of being congealed and sluggish, and this bile acts as a mild built-in laxative. The herb is also an alterative (blood purifying), anti-syphilitic, and tonic.

Cayenne *(Capsicum fastigiatum, Capsicum minimum or Capsicum annum)*
Cayenne is slightly laxative, stimulates the organs as it passes through, aids in rebuilding varicose conditions, and eliminates cholesterol from the area. Cayenne does a wonderful job of cleaning and rebuilding tissue.

Cascara Sagrada *(Rhamnus purshiana)*
This herb is called sacred bark and in small amounts, as used here, is a mild laxative. It is also a tonic for the peristaltic muscles, increases the secretions of the stomach, liver and pancreas, and is very remarkable in its action against torpor of the colon and constipation. It is unquestionably, one of the very best and safest laxatives ever discovered.

Ginger *(Zingiber officinalis)*
Its common name is Jamaican ginger. This herb is excellent for correcting flatulence. We need this herb to alleviate gas that is accumulated as the bile starts flowing into the intestines, mixing with old fecal matter and forming this condition. It is also an aid for relieving cramps and pains and for stimulating digestion.

Golden Seal *(Hydrastis canadensis)*
This wonderful herb is a tonic, mild laxative, alterative (for mucus membranes), antiseptic and antiemetic. It also kills infection, is a a blood purifier and aperient (mild laxative).

Lobelia *(Lobelia inflata)*
This is the accentuating herb that makes many of Dr. Christopher's formula work smoothly and efficiently. It is also an antispasmodic, a nervine, and will assist in cases of cramps and painful conditions.

Red Raspberry Leaves *(Rubus idaeus)*
This herb assists in supplying iron to the system in the form of citrate of iron. Upon this iron compound depends the remarkable blood making and regulating properties as well as the astringent and contracting action on the internal tissues and membranes. This herb is also hemostatic, antiseptic and antidiarrheal.

Turkey Rhubarb Root *(Rheum palmatum)*
Turkey (or China) rhubarb is such a mild aperient that it can be used for tiny babies because it gives smooth, easy, non-cramping bowel movements. This herb has many uses, it is a laxative, astringent, tonic, stomachic, brisk purgative and valuable in effecting a quick, safe emptying of the bowels. It does not clog or produce an "after-constipation" as so many cathartics do. It is especially useful in diarrhea caused by irritating substances in the intestines. It not only removes these substances, but its delayed astringent action helps control diarrhea.

Fennel *(Foeniculum officinale)*
This herb is noted for its relief in cases of flatulence in digestion, cramps and spasms, nausea, pin worms, and in hepatic conditions (liver, gall bladder malfunctions).

Each of these nine herbs has a specific job to do and combined, make an excellent herbal food for the small and large intestine. Because we have years of accumulated filth and fecal matter in our bowels, using this formula for nine months to a year or more, in some cases, is not severe at all. Working with both the mucusless diet and the Lower Bowel Formula, you can have easy bowel movements for the rest of your life. And if you continually observe the mucusless diet, soon no Lower Bowel Formula will be needed.

Remember, this herbal combination is not habit forming or one that you have to increase as time goes on, but one that works on the cause and not just as a laxative or flush for temporary relief. You can watch and regulate the amount of this Lower Bowel Formula and eventually reduce it until you have easy, regular bowel movements without the use of this aid at all. Your proper diet will help sustain regular movements.

During the first years of the Lower Bowel Formula's use, during the 1940s, people said that it was griping. For this reason, we added the ginger. Some asked, "Why not add an aid in the combination for the nausea that happened in a few cases?" So we added red raspberry leaves to relieve this condition and to add lost iron and fruit acids that were causing this problem.

Remember the important function of your bowel and give it the consistent nourishment and care it requires to keep the body clean and healthy. Constipation is the root of all *disease*, therefore, let us take time to exercise, correct our posture, drink plenty of distilled water and fresh juices, and eat wholesome living foods that will aid our bowels to serve us more perfectly.

Quick Colon Formula #1
Curacao and Cape Aloes (*Aloe vera*)
Senna Leaves and Pods (*Senna alexandrina*)
Cascara Sagrada Bark (*Rhamnus purshiana*)
Barberry Root Bark (*Berberis vulgaris*)
Ginger Root (*Zingiber officinale*)

Garlic Bulb (*Allium sativum*)
African Bird Pepper or Cayenne Pepper (*Capsicum spp.*)
This blend of herbs is a powerful laxative or purgative and was formulated for cases of extreme constipation. Because this formula is a pure laxative and does not feed the bowel, it is not intended for long term use. The normal dosage of this formula starts at one capsule once a day. The dosage increases one capsule each day until the desired results are achieved (two or three bowel movements a day). After these results are achieved, gradually switch to the Lower Bowel Formula for long term maintenance as needed.

Quick Colon Formula #2
Flax Seed (*Linum usitatissimum*)
Apple Fruit Pectin (*Malus spp.*)
Bentonite Clay
Psyllium Seed and Husk (*Plantago ovata, Plantago ispaghula*)
Slippery Elm Inner Bark (*Ulmus rubra*)
Marshmallow Root (*Althea officinalis*)
Fennel Seed (*Foeniculum vulgare*)
Activated Willow Charcoal
If a deeper colon cleanse is needed, this formula can be used in conjunction with Quick Colon Formula #1. This formula was designed to pull toxins and deposits out of the colon and eliminate them from the body. This formula is slightly constipating and should not be taken without Quick Colon Formula #1. Also, because of the cleansing nature of this formula, it should be taken with large amounts of water and only when the bowels are regular (two or three bowel movements a day). Directions: Mix one heaping teaspoon of powder with four to six ounces of fresh juice or water. After consumption, drink an additional eight or sixteen ounces of liquid (preferably water). Repeat five times a day until finished with the bottle. The Quick Colon Formula #2 is not intended for long term use.

Sunflower Leaf Tea (*Helianthus spp.*)

Sunflower leaf tea should only be used in cases of severe dehydration and diarrhea. It stops diarrhea within a short period of time. Usually only a small amount (i.e. a half a cup) is needed to accomplish this.

Three Day Cleanse

Dr. Christopher's book *The Three Day Cleanse and Mucusless Diet*, has helped many people with severe health problems. The three day juice and water fast described in this book removes toxins from the blood stream, liver and bowel. Dr. Christopher also explains which foods are mucus forming and how mucus forming foods need to be eliminated from the diet to achieve optimum health. Fasting only with water is not recommended, because it causes the body to flush out toxins faster than the body can handle. The three day cleanse that Dr. Christopher recommended eliminates toxins in a way the body can handle while giving it enough energy to remain active.

Turmeric (*Curcuma longa*)

Clinical evidence indicates that *Curcuma longa* (Turmeric) has strong antiinflammatory and antispasmodic effects in the intestinal tract[8]. One of the herb's active ingredients (curcumin) acts as a nonsteroidal antiinflammatory, helpful for easing a spastic colon and calming colitis and many other intestinal complaints. It also is a natural pain reliever, with an action much like cayenne pepper.

"Indigestion is charged by God with enforcing morality on the stomach."
—*Victor Hugo*

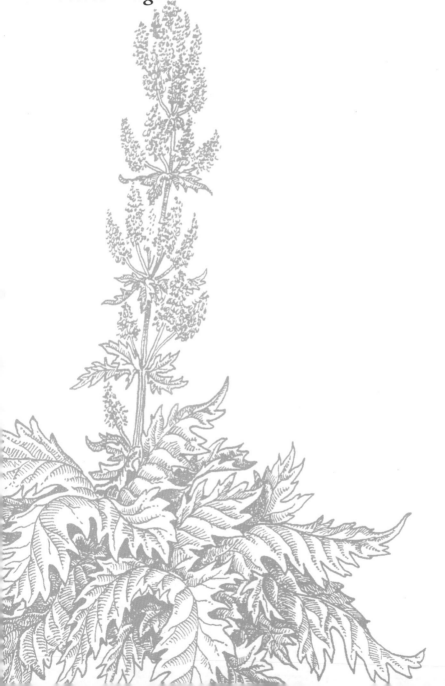

Chapter 4:
Digestive Diseases

The following is a list of diseases along with their herbal and natural healing protocols. These therapies and formulas were used by Dr. Christopher in his practice and have proven themselves to be safe and effective for most people. You can find descriptions of each therapy in the previous chapter. As always, when dealing with a serious medical issue it is vitally important to get an accurate diagnosis before considering any treatment.

Appendicitis

Appendicitis is inflammation of the appendix, a small pouch attached to the cecum which is the beginning of the large intestine. The appendix is located in the lower right side of the abdomen. Over 250,000 people are hospitalized each year with appendicitis. If left untreated, an inflamed appendix may burst, causing infection. Serious infections can lead to death if not treated properly. Because of the risk of rupture and infection, appendicitis is considered an emergency and should be treated by a competent healer. The symptoms of appendicitis include pain in the right side of the abdomen often under and to the right of the navel, nausea, vomiting, constipation, diarrhea, inability to pass gas, a low fever that begins after other symptoms occur, abdominal swelling, or pain that increases when moving, taking deep breaths, coughing, sneezing, or being touched in the area. A sharp and sudden pain or a sudden increase in temperature may indicate that the appendix has burst. Extra care should be taken if this occurs. A burst appendix may release its infectious contents into the abdominal cavity causing systemic infection and shock. Remember, the appendix is an important part of the immune system and should only be surgically removed as a last resort.

Appendicitis Protocol

This is a twenty-four hour a day treatment. Several people may perform this protocol in shifts even while the sufferer is sleeping. The therapies that follow may be performed in any order (some may not be necessary in every case.)

1. A liquid only diet (solid food may compound the problem). Teas, including catnip and fennel, comfrey, and chamomile are helpful. Onion garlic soup with a little olive oil may also be used. Fresh papaya and pineapple juices contain enzymes that help break down deposits in the intestines. These juices may be used if needed. Another liquid therapy that may be used is the following: Blend 4 Tbs of olive oil, 16oz of grapefruit juice, and 4 cloves of fresh garlic together and consume twice a day. This mixture is soothing, antibiotic, nutritive, and helps protect the body from the toxic accumulation in the colon.

2. Castor oil fomentations should be applied to the appendix area along with hot and cold applications. Let the sufferer tell you when to change from hot to cold. When the fomentation will become uncomfortable it is a signal indicating that it's time to switch from hot to cold or vice-versa.

3. Very light abdominal massage over the appendix area and then slightly deeper up the ascending colon and along the transverse colon moving away from the appendix (again let the sufferer be your guide on how deep to massage). Follow instructions on page 36.

4. Reflexology over the lower bowel reflex areas, going lightly over the appendix area and a bit deeper moving away from the appendix. See the reflexology chart on page 53.

5. The Lower Bowel Formula should be used. Start out with a moderate amount and increase from there.

6. A low volume enema of catnip and fennel to ease cramping and pain. Be careful not to use too much liquid in the enema. Excess pressure in the bowel may cause complications.

7. In case of infection or rupture of the appendix, take X-Ceptic by mouth along with echinacea, X-Ceptic can also be used externally as a rub over the site of the infection.

8. Use hydrotherapy in a shower or tub. In a tub of hot water, apply hot and cold packs to the appendix area.

9. Pain medication should be avoided at all costs. Pain is a signal that something in the body needs to be addressed as soon as possible. Often pain will tell you how the therapy is proceeding and what to do next. Lobelia tincture is helpful in many cases of severe pain. Apply lobelia tincture over the area while doing the light abdominal massage, reflexology or hot and cold packs.

10. Kloss' Appendicitis Poultice. Mix one Tbs. lobelia powder, a large handful of crushed mullein leaves, and a sprinkle of ginger root powder. Mix with water and slippery elm and apply as a paste over the appendix site. Use hot and cold packs on top of the paste.

Celiac Disease
Celiac disease is a digestive disorder that affects the small intestine and interferes with absorption of nutrients from food. People who have celiac disease have a low tolerance for a protein called gluten, which is found in wheat, rye, barley, and possibly oats. When people with celiac disease eat foods

containing gluten, their immune system attacks cells in the small intestine. Specifically, tiny fingerlike protrusions, called villi, on the lining of the small intestine are affected. Nutrients from food are absorbed into the bloodstream through these villi. Without villi, a person becomes malnourished—regardless of the quantity of food eaten. Because the body's own immune system causes the damage, celiac disease is considered an autoimmune disorder. However, it is also classified as a disease of malabsorption because nutrients are not absorbed. Celiac disease is also known as celiac sprue, nontropical sprue, and gluten-sensitive enteropathy.

Celiac disease occurs when gluten protein is introduced into the blood stream without being broken down properly by the digestive system. There are several circumstances where this can happen. One of the most common is when something has compromised the integrity of the intestinal wall and has caused it to bleed into the digestive tract. Proteins pass through this opening and enter the blood stream, sensitizing the immune system. The immune cells remember the protein and react strongly when exposed to it again.

Celiac disease affects people differently. Some develop symptoms as children, others as adults. One factor that may play a role in when and how celiac appears is whether and how long a person was breast-fed—the longer one was breast-fed, the less likely a person is to develop celiac disease. The introduction of wheat protein (as well as other grain proteins) into a child's diet before they can be properly digested may sensitize them to the protein and make them more susceptible to this disease.

Symptoms of celiac disease may seem unrelated to the bowel and are often misdiagnosed. They may include any of the following: recurring abdominal bloating and pain, chronic diarrhea, weight loss, pale, foul-smelling stool, unexplained anemia (low count of red blood cells), recurring flatulence, bone pain, behavior changes (including depression and irritability), muscle cramps, fatigue, delayed growth, failure to thrive in infants, painful joints, seizures, tingling numbness in the legs (from nerve damage), pale sores inside the mouth (called aphthus ulcers), painful skin rash (called dermatitis herpetiformis), tooth discoloration or loss of enamel, missed menstrual periods (often because of excessive weight loss).

Useful therapies include: Slippery elm and licorice root gruel, juice therapy, Immucalm, Vitalerbs, abdominal massage, the Lower Bowel Formula, and a gluten free diet.

Colic

Colic is severe abdominal pain that usually only occurs in small infants. According to the American Academy of Pediatrics, of the almost 4,000,000 babies born in the United States each year, one in four will develop colic at some time. One of the biggest factors leading to colic is lactose intolerance. The nursing mother may have dairy in her diet or is giving the infant a dairy milk based formula. The proteins in dairy milk (as well as other man made milk substitutes) are hard to the infant's immature digestive tract to process. This causes the stomach upset known as colic. There are also other factors that lead to colic but the treatment is the same. Symptoms of colic include a hard and distended belly, legs and arms drawn up and the fists clenched, coldness in the hands and feet.

Useful therapies include: Stopping all dairy consumption, Catnip and Fennel tea (for the mother), Kid-e-Col for the child, light abdominal massage, light reflexology, warm compress over the stomach, massage with a small amount of lobelia tincture over the stomach and diaphragm area.

Colitis or Ulcerative Colitis

Ulcerative colitis is a disease that is characterized by inflammation and sores (ulcers) in the top layers in the lining of the large intestine. The inflammation usually occurs in the rectum and lower part of the colon, but it may affect the entire colon. Ulcerative colitis rarely affects the small intestine except for the lower section, called the ileum. Ulcerative colitis may also be called colitis, or ileitis. The inflammation makes the colon empty frequently, causing diarrhea. Ulcers form in places where the inflammation has killed cells that line the colon; the ulcers bleed and produce pus and mucus. Over 275,000 people are hospitalized with colitis each year. Two of the biggest factors contributing to the high incidence of colitis and ulcerative conditions are poor diet and the use of nonsteroidal anti-inflammatories. The standard American diet is low fiber, high in fat, and void of fruits, grains, vegetables, nuts, and seeds. With this kind of constant abuse, its no wonder that so many people have swollen ulcerated colons. Nonsteroidal anti-inflammatories create localized inflammation in the stomach, and intestine, after a few uses this inflammation can develop into sores on the intestinal wall and eventually ulcers. Thousands of people die each year from bleeding ulcers caused by these harmful drugs.

Useful therapies include: Slippery elm and licorice root gruel, juice therapy, abdominal massage, cayenne pepper, and the Lower Bowel Formula.

Colon-Rectal Cancer

This is one of the most prevalent forms of cancer in the United States today. 133,000 new cases are diagnosed and over 55,000 people die each year from this disease. Lack of high fiber foods such as vegetables, fruit, grains, nuts, and seeds as well as too many highly constipating foods such as meat, white flour, sugar, and dairy products has made colon-rectal cancer the killer it is today. Cancer is a sign that the eliminative channels are blocked and a toxic condition exists throughout the body (not just in the organ where the cancer is). Cancer can be cut out, burned out, or poisoned out of the body, but the environment that caused the cancer is still there. The cause of the disease must be addressed. For this reason, we cleanse the lower bowel, the liver and gallbladder, the kidneys, and the blood stream. When these organs are functioning properly, the body has an easier time defeating cancer.

Useful therapies include: The mucusless diet, the Lower

71

Bowel Formula, castor oil fomentations, the Blood Stream Formula (Red Clover Combination), apricot seeds, slippery elm and licorice root gruel, as well as the Three Day Cleanse.

Constipation

Constipation occurs when the bowel becomes blocked with old fecal matter and fails to move at least twice a day. Diarrhea is another symptom of constipation. When the bowel is constipated, the body will attempt to "flush out" the blockage with water. The result is watery stools or diarrhea. Factors that contribute to constipation include eating mucus forming foods, not enough fiber in the diet, not enough liquids (especially distilled water), lack of exercise, pharmaceutical medications, irritable bowel syndrome, changes in life or routine (such as pregnancy, older age, and travel), ignoring the urge to have a bowel movement, specific diseases such as multiple sclerosis and lupus, or problems with the colon and rectum. Constipation is responsible for over 2,000,000 doctor visits each year and over 100,000 hospitalizations each year.

Useful therapies include: The Lower Bowel Formula, a high fiber diet, rebounding, regular exercise, drinking more water, reflexology, and abdominal massage. In severe cases use the Quick Colon Formula #1, enemas, or colonics may be used to overcome the constipation and then continue with the Lower Bowel Formula as long as necessary. The papaya cleanse may also be used if the constipation is caused by old blockages.

Dyspepsia (see indigestion)

Diarrhea

As mentioned previously, chronic diarrhea is really an advanced form of constipation. The body is attempting to "flush out" hardened fecal matter with a lot of liquid. In these cases it is best to use soothing herbs that add bulk to a bowel movement. In cases of acute diarrhea caused by a stomach infection or food poisoning the body is attempting to rid itself of the offending food, virus, or bacteria. It is important to let the body do what comes naturally and only stop diarrhea in an emergency. It is also important to keep the body hydrated with plenty of distilled water and fresh fruit and vegetable juices.

Useful therapies include: Distilled water, juice therapy, slippery elm and licorice root gruel, abdominal massage, castor oil packs, and the Lower Bowel Formula. In cases of severe dehydration use a small amount of sunflower tea. This will stop diarrhea a within a short period of time.

Diverticulitis

Over 2,000,000 Americans each year are diagnosed with diverticulitis. Those with this disease have small pouches in their colons that bulge outward through weak spots, like an inner tube that pokes through weak places in an old tire. Each pouch is called a diverticulum. Pouches (plural) are called diverticula. The condition of having diverticula is called diverticulosis. More than half of all Americans age 60 to 80, and almost everyone over age 80, have diverticulosis. Diverticulitis occurs when diverticula become infected or inflamed. This happens when mucus, stool, and bacteria are caught in the diverticula causing irritation. An attack of diverticulitis can develop suddenly and without warning. Diverticulitis is common in developed or industrialized countries, particularly the United States, England, and Australia, where low-fiber, high mucus forming diets are common. The disease is rare in countries of Asia and Africa, where people eat high-fiber vegetable diets.

Useful therapies include: The Three Day Cleanse, the Lower Bowel Formula, abdominal massage, psyllium, the papaya diet, and castor oil fomentations.

Fissures (anal) and Anal Fistulas

An anal fissure is a small tear or cut in the skin lining the anus and lower rectum which can cause pain, discomfort, and/or bleeding. Anal fissures may be acute (recent) or chronic (present for a long time or recurring frequently). An acute

Colon Diseases

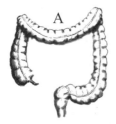

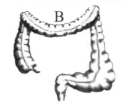

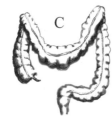

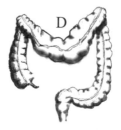

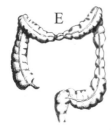

A. Healthy Colon
B. Colitis
C. Prolapsed Transverse Colon
D. Destended Transverse Colon
E. Spastic Colon

Colon Cross Sections

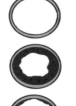 Healthy Colon

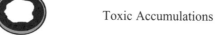 Toxic Accumulations

 Diverticula

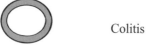 Colitis

fissure is usually due to constipation or hard bowel movements, while a chronic fissure may be either due to a lifetime of poor bowel habits, overly tight or spastic anal sphincter muscles. Symptoms may include the presence of red blood in the stool, pain when having a bowel movement, itchy anus, pain between bowel movements. Those who have Crohn's Disease, and other colon diseases are more likely to develop anal fissures. An anal fistula is an abnormal track or channel from the anus that opens onto the skin surrounding the anus. Anal fistulas are caused by infection and abscess (collection of pus) in one of the glands near to the anus.

Useful therapies include: The Lower Bowel Formula, slippery elm and licorice root gruel, cayenne pepper, Complete Tissue Formula used as an enema or ointment, and juice therapy (especially cabbage and carrot).

Flatulence (gas)

Gas is normally present in the digestive tract, it comes from bacteria that helps break down food in your intestines. In cases of constipation, stress, or foods that are hard to digest (like dairy), gas may become a problem.

Useful therapies include: The Lower Bowel Formula, papaya and pineapple juice, abdominal massage, and catnip and fennel tea or extract.

Hemorrhoids

The term hemorrhoids refers to a condition in which the veins around the anus or lower rectum become varicose (swollen or inflamed). Hemorrhoids may result from straining to have a bowel movement or excess pressure in the lower abdomen. Contributing factors include pregnancy, aging, chronic constipation, diarrhea, or poor nutrition. Hemorrhoids are either inside the anus (internal) or under the skin around the anus (external). Hemorrhoids usually are not dangerous or life threatening. Although many people have hemorrhoids, not all experience symptoms. The most common symptom of internal hemorrhoids include bright red blood covering the stool, on toilet paper, or in the toilet bowl, itchy anus, and presence of a swollen vein. However, an internal hemorrhoid may protrude through the anus outside the body, becoming irritated and painful. This is known as a protruding hemorrhoid.

Symptoms of external hemorrhoids may include painful swelling or a hard lump around the anus that results when a blood clot forms. This condition is known as a thrombosed external hemorrhoid. In addition, excessive straining, rubbing, or cleaning around the anus may cause irritation with bleeding and/or itching, which may produce a vicious cycle of symptoms.

Useful therapies include: The mucusless diet, the Lower Bowel Formula, white oak bark fomentation on the affected area, Complete Tissue Formula ointment applied topically between bowel movements, and cold aloe vera gel applied topically. Hemorrhoid sufferers often lack Vitamin C and bioflavonoids in their diets; fresh citrus juice and small amounts of cayenne pepper are some of the most effective remedies for chronic problems.

Indigestion

Acid indigestion, also known as upset stomach, heartburn, or dyspepsia is characterized by discomfort or a burning feeling in the upper abdomen, often accompanied by nausea, abdominal bloating, belching, and sometimes vomiting. Indigestion might be caused by a disease in the digestive tract, but for many people, it is caused by eating too much, eating too quickly, eating high-fat foods, or eating during stressful situations. Smoking, drinking alcohol, drinking soda or coffee, using medications that irritate the stomach lining, being tired, and having ongoing stress can also cause indigestion or make it worse. Some people have persistent indigestion that is not related to any of these factors. This type of indigestion is called functional or non-ulcer dyspepsia, and may be caused by a problem in the muscular squeezing action of the stomach.

Useful therapies include: The mucusless diet, slippery elm and licorice root gruel, abdominal massage, rebounding, reflexology, and Catnip and Fennel or Kid-e-Col.

Irritable Bowel Syndrome

Irritable bowel syndrome (IBS) is a fairly common disorder of the intestines that affects over 5,000,000 people each year. Its symptoms are cramping, pain, flatulence, bloating, and changes in bowel habits. Some people with IBS have constipation, others have diarrhea, and some people experience both. Sometimes the person with IBS has cramping and an urge to move the bowels but cannot do so. In IBS, the bowel becomes hypersensitive and spasms. These spasms can be brought about by foods such as dairy products, wheat and corn fractions, and meat consumption. Stress, pharmaceutical drugs, and alcohol may also trigger these intestinal spasms in those who are sensitive. This condition is the result of a poor diet, and stressful lifestyle.

Useful therapies include: Immuncalm, slippery elm and licorice root gruel, and dietary changes. Small nutritious meals along with fresh juices are recommended. Reducing stress and anxiety are also important.

Leaky Gut Syndrome

This condition occurs when undigested protein enters from the digestive tract into the blood stream wreaking havoc with the immune system. Protein may enter into the bloodstream either because it has been poorly digested or there is an opening in the digestive tract allowing blood to enter and intestinal contents to leak out into circulation. The immune system recognizes the protein as an invader and attacks it. The immune system then remembers the invader and produces antibodies to it. Sometimes these foreign proteins look like our own proteins, and the body attacks itself. The result is an autoimmune disorder. Foods that may cause leaky gut syndrome include alcohol, dairy, processed foods, fried foods, and processed grains. Other factors that may contribute to leaky gut syndrome include intestinal infection, candida infection, parasite infection, and use of pharmaceutical

77

medication (especially aspirin, ibuprofen, and antibiotics).

Useful therapies include: Juice therapy (especially cabbage and carrot), Immucalm, slippery elm and licorice root gruel, and abdominal massage.

Polyps

The word polyp refers to any overgrowth of tissue from the surface of mucous membranes (such as nasal, esophageal, and intestinal polyps). Intestinal polyps grow out of the lining of the small and large intestines (including the rectum) and dangle into the intestinal opening. Polyps come in a variety of shapes and often grow stalks which make them more troublesome.

Polyps of the colon and rectum are usually benign and produce no symptoms (asymptomatic), but they may cause painless rectal bleeding. Large polyps may eventually cause intestinal obstruction, which produces cramping abdominal pain with nausea and vomiting. There may be single or multiple polyps and they become more common as people age. Some conditions cause a blanket of small polyps on the intestinal wall that can interfere with absorption of nutrients. Over time, certain types of polyps, called adenomas, can develop into cancer. Adenomas are present in thirty percent of all adults over the age of fifty. Polyps greater than one centimeter have a greater cancer risk associated with them than polyps under one centimeter. Risk factors for intestinal polyps include advancing age, cigarette smoking, high-fat or low-fiber diet, obesity, and a family history of polyps.

Useful therapies include: The Lower Bowel Formula, the Blood Stream Formula, a low-fat high-fiber diet, slippery elm and licorice root gruel, and the Complete Tissue Formula. Apricot seeds may also be a useful therapy if the condition is cancerous or precancerous.

Pregnancy and Nursing

Although pregnancy is not a disease, it is a condition that often causes constipation. Special care should be taken not to put the pregnancy at risk in any way. Nursing mothers also need to take care because what they eat and the supplements they take will affect their child. For this reason we suggest only the most gentle treatments be used on a pregnant or nursing mothers. When taking any herbal supplement, these women should take the lowest recommended dose and the safest product available.

Useful therapies include: The Lower Bowel Formula, slippery elm and licorice root gruel, fresh fruit, and dried prunes and apricots. Many have found ginger to be the best remedy for morning sickness and nausea that often accompany pregnancy.

Prolapsed Bowel

When the colon (especially the transverse colon) is chronically constipated and swollen, it will often hang downwards. If this condition persists a bloated and heavy colon may crowd the other organs of the abdomen including the urinary bladder, uterus, and rectum. A prolapsed bowel can cause other organs to become prolapsed, and constipated also. This condition often causes the abdomen to protrude giving the appearance of a "pot" or "beer" belly.

Useful therapies include: The Lower Bowel Formula, abdominal massage, rebounding, a high fiber diet, and juice fasting. In extreme cases it may be useful to administer a colonic or high enema to dissolve constipated fecal matter.

Reflux Disease, Hiatal Hernia, and Heartburn

Gastroesophageal reflux disease (GERD) is a digestive disorder that affects the lower esophageal sphincter (LES)—the muscle connecting the esophagus with the stomach. This muscle closes off the stomach, allowing food to enter but protecting the esophagus from its acidic contents. When pressure is placed on the stomach because of pregnancy, poor posture, obesity, or a sedentary lifestyle, the LES is strained open and the esophagus is exposed to the stomach's contents. A Hiatal hernia occurs when the upper part of the stomach is forced through an opening in the diaphragm. This will also cause the LES to stay open.

Heartburn (also called acid indigestion), is the most common symptom of both GERD and Hiatal hernia. Heartburn usually feels like a burning chest pain beginning behind the breastbone and moving upward to the neck and throat. More than sixty million American adults experience GERD and heartburn at least once a month, and about 25,000,000 adults suffer daily from heartburn. Twenty-five percent of pregnant women experience daily heartburn, and more than fifty percent have occasional symptoms. The most common medication for these diseases is antacids. These acid reducing treatments may stop the symptoms for a while but do not address the cause and may even make the problem worse. When the stomach's acidic environment is reduced it will begin to produce more acid. In response to the acid, more antacid is taken, and the injurious chain continues. The body depends on the stomach's acid to break down proteins and kill bacteria, if this important part of the digestive process is blocked, many diseases may result including candida, autoimmune problems, intestinal infections, malabsorption, Crohn's Disease, irritable bowel syndrome, and colitis.

Useful therapies include: Exercise, slippery elm and licorice root gruel, ginger, abdominal massage, rebounding, and juice therapy.

Stomachache and Upset Stomach

Most childhood (and adult) stomachaches come from stress. Whether it is school, work, or socially related, tension can cause the stomach to ache. Soothing and stress reducing herbs generally do a great job at relieving these stomach complaints. If the symptoms persist or if they are accompanied by vomiting or diarrhea then the stomachache may be a symptom of something else including ulcers, irritable bowel syndrome, and gastric infection.

Useful therapies include: Kid-e-Col, Catnip and Fennel tea (or Kid-e-Col), ginger (for nausea), kava (for anxiety), Kid-e-Trac (for emotional clarity), and stress relieving activities.

Ulcers (Gastric and Duodenal)

During normal digestion, food moves from the mouth down the esophagus into the stomach. The stomach produces hydrochloric acid and an enzyme called pepsin to digest the food. From the stomach, food passes into the upper part of the small intestine, called the duodenum, where digestion and nutrient absorption continue.

An ulcer is a sore or lesion that forms in the lining of the stomach or duodenum. Ulcers in the stomach are called gastric or stomach ulcers. Those in the duodenum are called duodenal ulcers. In general, ulcers in the stomach and duodenum are referred to as peptic ulcers. These conditions affect over 5,000,000 people each year.

Factors that contribute to peptic ulcers include dairy consumption, heavy meat consumption, stress, and many pharmaceutical medications. Thousands of people die every year from taking nonsteroidal antiinflammatories like aspirin and ibuprofen. These drugs cause local irritation in the mucus lining of the gastrointestinal tract. Repeated abuse of these drugs causes ulcers that may bleed uncontrollably.

Doctors and scientists now suspect the bacteria Helicobacter pylori (*H. pylori*) as the cause of many ulcerative conditions and are treating them with antibiotics. In reality diet and lifestyle create the environment for this and other bacteria to thrive. Although *H. pylori* are found in many of those who have peptic ulcers, they are a symptom and not the cause of peptic ulcers.

Useful therapies include: Slippery elm and licorice root gruel, dietary and lifestyle changes, peppermint tea, cayenne pepper (to control bleeding and soothe the gastrointestinal tract), cabbage and carrot juice, and reflexology.

Ninety Percent of all disease is caused by constipation

Many students are surprised when we say that over ninety percent of all disease is caused by constipation. Even diseases that seem unrelated such as eczema, depression, and backache are often caused by a toxic and overloaded bowel. The intestines function as the "sewer system" of the body. They eliminate wastes from almost every organ including the liver, gallbladder, pancreas, blood stream, lymph, and brain. When this "sewer" is backed up or isn't functioning properly, the other organs cannot eliminate their wastes. The result is not only a constipated bowel but constipated organs throughout the body that become diseased and exhibit almost any symptom. Below is a list of a few common diseases and how they are related to constipation:

Eczema, acne, and other skin problems:

The liver acts like a garbage collector for the blood stream. It filters out toxins from digestion, excess hormones, old blood cells, and anything that shouldn't be in the bloodstream. If the liver cannot eliminate these toxins efficiently because the bowel is constipated, a myriad of health problems may result. The body will often use the skin to eliminate toxins—the result is skin diseases. These skin conditions can be treated with the Lower Bowel Formula and the Liver Gallbladder Formula.

Depression, anxiety, and attention deficit disorder:

Emotions are both electrical and chemical in nature. When neuro-chemicals and hormones are not eliminated by the liver because the bowel and liver are constipated, they recirculate and cause emotional disturbances. Manic depression can often be eliminated when the liver and bowel are cleansed and working properly. Hyperactivity and attention deficit disorder are often cured by changing the diet and making sure the bowel is eliminating properly.

Backache, menstrual pain, and prostate problems:
The organs of the abdomen are situated very close together and even share circulation with one another. When the lower bowel becomes blocked, the toxic condition can spread to nearby organs and structures including the uterus, prostate, lower back, and sciatic nerve. This toxic condition can cause almost any disease.

Heart disease, high cholesterol:
The heart and circulatory system rely on a clean blood stream for it to properly function. If the bowel is constipated there is no way for waste including cholesterol to be eliminated. The result is high cholesterol and waste in the blood stream with nowhere to go. This waste ends up collecting on the walls of arteries throughout the body raising blood pressure and causing blockages, strokes and other problems.

Infertility, hormonal problems, premature aging, and malnourishment:
When the intestine is clogged and coated with old matter, it does not allow many nutrients to pass through its walls. This can cause a state of malnourishment throughout the body. When this happens the body doesn't have the proper nutrients to create hormones, build a strong circulatory system, repair broken bones, or repair the thousands of microscopic damages that happen everyday. As damage goes un-repaired because of this lack of nutrients the body starts degenerating, we start feeling older and looking older, our bodies stop working how they should, and we feel tired and run down.

"Without proper diet, medicine is of no use. With proper diet, medicine is of no need"
—*Ancient Ayurvedic Proverb*

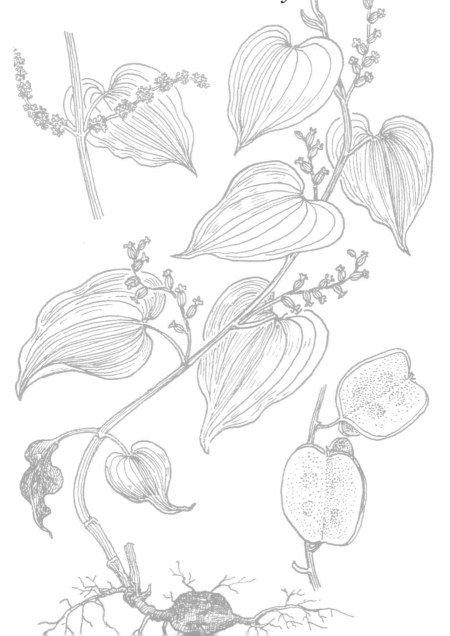

Chapter 5
Foods that Kill and Foods that Heal

What not to eat

Imagine that your body is a new car designed to last a long time (we used this analogy in the beginning of this book). In the owners manual that came with the car, the manufacturer describes the kind of fuel that should be used, how often the filters need to be replaced, when to change the oil and other fluids, and when to schedule tune-ups. The manual claims that if you follow its directions, you will have a pleasant worry free ownership and enjoy the car for years to come. But if you fail to take care of the car as directed, problems will result and you will have to pay for costly repairs. Our bodies are very much like new cars when we are born. If taken care of properly, our bodies can be healthy for a long time without much worry. When we eat the wrong foods, don't exercise, and don't take care of ourselves, our bodies break down, and we have to repair them.

According to the United States' Department of Agriculture, the average American diet consists of almost two hundred pounds of meat, hundreds of gallons of milk (in the form of milk, cheese, and milk solids), and over one hundred and seventy pounds of sugar per person each year. If the human body had an owners manual, is this the kind of fuel it would want us to use? These foods clog up our filters (liver), engine (heart), and fuel system (pancreas, circulatory and digestive systems). It's no wonder Americans have extremely high rates of obesity, diabetes, heart disease, and intestinal disorders. This diet is the reason modern America is the most constipated society in the history of the world.

One of the least understood aspects of human physiology is the role mucus plays in our digestive system. Our digestive tract is lined with mucus membrane. This tissue produces a thin layer of mucus that serves many functions. It traps food particles that need to be digested, it is home to the intestinal flora, it protects the intestinal wall from damage, and it acts as a lubricant for the digestive system. Mucus is essential to the health of our bodies. Only a thin layer of mucus is needed to serve this function. Some food causes our bodies to produce excess mucus. This overproduction of mucus can accumulate almost anywhere in the body including the sinuses, bowel, lungs, and many organs. When mucus accumulates it slows the normal functions of the body (constipates) and provides a home for unfriendly bacteria. Producing an abundance of mucus may be the body's reaction to a perceived toxin. When the body encounters a potential threat it creates a barrier of mucus to protect itself. When the body is constantly exposed to this threat, the mucus builds up, creating an unhealthy environment.

The following "foods" cause our bodies to create excess mucus:

White flour: white breads, pastries, most prepared bread products, donuts, pasta, and crackers. These foods act like paste in the digestive system, slowing down digestion and gluing material to the intestinal walls.

Sugar: breakfast cereals, carbonated drinks, many bottled and frozen drinks, most desserts, canned fruit, syrup, ice cream, and most snack foods. Substances such as table sugar and high fructose corn syrup should be classified as harmful drugs. They cause the pancreas to work overtime as well as provide the perfect environment for bacterial to grow in.

Dairy: milk, cheese, cottage cheese, cream, goat milk, any food that contains milk or whey solids, cream soups, and most prepared foods. Humans are the only animal that drink milk after they are weaned. This unnatural practice is responsible for much of the disease in modern societies.

Additives: foods with dyes, flavor enhancers, monosodium glutamate, anti-caking agents, preservatives, chemicals, non organic vitamins and minerals, and artificial flavors. These substances have been linked to hyperactivity, multiple chemical sensitivity syndrome, and many other illnesses.

Meat: beef, pork, chicken, turkey, and fish. Meat is hard to digest and often putrefies before it leaves the body. This "second hand" protein often carries with it the toxins, and microorganisms from the animal it was made from. Organ meat, beef, and pork, are especially harmful and should be avoided.

The more a food is cooked the more mucus-forming and constipating it becomes. Raw food when well chewed provides living enzymes, and organic vitamins and minerals that can be fully assimilated by the body. When food is cooked, the enzymes start breaking down, the vitamins and minerals become inorganic and the food becomes less healthy. When food is fully cooked it is totally dead and unwholesome. You cannot build a healthy living body with dead food. If you want to know if your food is dead or not, plant it. If properly watered and cared for it should sprout within a few days. If it doesn't sprout, you know the food was not living, and not wholesome.

What you should eat

Many people look at the list above and cry "You're taking away all my food, what is there left to eat?" They have been raised their whole lives on dead foods and have no idea what delicious alternatives exist. Millions of recipes have been created using whole foods such as fruits, grains, vegetables, nuts, and seeds. Recipe books, raw food and vegetarian restaurants, raw food classes, and support groups have made it easier than ever to eat well. Even organic food is appearing in supermarkets, health food stores, and farmer's markets all over the country. Listed below are some healthful, and appealing dishes made with raw and living foods. These recipes can be found in _Living in the Raw_ by Rose Lee Calabro.

Tripple Berry Ice Cream

Apple Walnut Pie

Curried Grain

Vegetable Lasagna

Marinated Fava Beans

Mexican Stuffed Peppers

Lemony Tufu Pate'

Veggie Burgers

Apricot Quinoa Salad

Creamy Garlic Dressing

Garlic Herb Dressing

Carrot Curry Soup

Stuffed Mushrooms with Pine Nuts and Basil

Apricot Almond Low Heat Bread

Low Heat Cinnamon Date Bread

Banana Nut Cream Torte

Strawberry Mousse

Pinwheel Cake

Carob Truffles

Ice Candy

Almond Orange Cookies

Banana Nut Cookies

Fudge Brownies

Therapeutic Foods

Hippocrates said "Let your food be your medicine and your medicine be your food." In other words, food can be used to heal your body, not just feed it. Some of these therapeutic foods for the digestive system are listed below:

Demulcent foods such as avocados and okra, soothe inflamed tissue and provide nutrients to rebuild damaged mucus membrane. Demulcent foods are helpful in cases of Crohn's Disease, irritable bowel syndrome, anal fissures, colitis, and ulcers.

Enzyme rich foods like papaya and pineapple, help the body break down food and eliminate old deposits in the intestines. These foods are helpful in cases of obstructed bowel problems, constipation, and malabsorption of food.

Astringent foods such as pomegranates, rhubarb, choke cherries, and many herbal teas help the body reduce bleeding in the digestive tract and control diarrhea. They also slow the flow of secretions into the digestive tract when needed.

Fibrous fruits and vegetables such as broccoli, cauliflower, figs, dates, and prunes act as gentle laxatives, scrubbing the sides of the digestive tract and adding bulk to bowel movements. They are gentle enough for children and have the added benefit of lowering the rate of colon-rectal cancer.

Sour foods like lemons, limes, and vinegar stimulate the appetite, improve digestion, and encourage the production of saliva which helps break down carbohydrates. Natural sour foods help alkalinize the body, making it healthier.

Bitter foods like dandelion greens, endive, and parsley, stimulate the production of bile which aids the body in digesting fats. They also help the liver filter toxins out of the blood. Bitter foods are beneficial for many diseases including depression, skin problems, and liver conditions. In Europe, it is popular to drink daily bitters (a drink with bitter herbs) in order to stimulate the digestive tract. Animals in the wild naturally seek out bitter foods as part of their daily diet.

Pungent foods such as horseradish, garlic, onions and cayenne stimulate the entire digestive system. They also act as natural antibiotics and antiseptics in the stomach and bowels. Pungent foods stimulate the stomach to digest more efficiently and trigger the body to get rid of excess mucus.

Fermented foods like sauerkraut, kimchi, rejuvalac, and

vinegar help replenish and balance intestinal flora. This is especially helpful in cases of recurrent diarrhea and candida.

A classic example of therapeutic foods is this recipe for prune pudding. Prunes are a fibrous and demulcent food that lend themselves well as a treatment for constipation. This tasty recipe is especially useful for children, but adults love it too.

Norwegian Prune Pudding
1/2 pound prunes
2 cups hot water
1/3 cup honey
1/8 teaspoon salt
1/2 teaspoon cinnamon
1/2 cup boiling water
1/3 cup cornstarch or arrow root
1/4 cup cold water
1 Tablespoon lemon juice

Place the prunes in a saucepan, cover with hot water and let stand for one hour. Place over low heat and simmer until soft. Remove the pits, then return the prunes to the cooking water. Add honey, salt, cinnamon, and boiling water. Simmer ten minutes. Mix cornstarch or arrow root with cold water to make a smooth paste. Add to prune mixture and cook for five minutes, stirring constantly. Add lemon juice. Pour into a large serving dish and chill. May be served with soy cream or soy milk
Yield: 6 Servings

References:

[1] Gastric secretory function in peptic ulcer in youth and the effect on it of diet therapyVopr Pitan (Russian). 1977 Jul-Aug;(4):57-63

[2] Chili protects against aspirin-induced gastroduodenal mucosal injury in humans. Digest of Digestive Science. 1995 Mar;40(3):580-3. By Yeoh KG, Kang JY, Yap I, Guan R, Tan CC, Wee A, Teng.

[3] Protection against Helicobacter pylori and other bacterial infections by garlic. Journal of Nutrition. 2001 Mar;131(3s):1106S-8S

[4] The use of ginger (Zingiber officinale) as a potential antiinflammatory and anti-thrombotic agent. Prostaglandins and Essential Fatty Acids. 2002 Dec;67(6):475-8.

[5] Effects of ginger on motion sickness and gastric slow-wave dysrhythmias induced by circular vection. American Journal of Gastrointestinal and Liver Physiology. 2003 Mar;284(3):G481-9.

[6] Effects of biologically active food additives on digestive function in experimental lead and chromium poisoning Gig Sanit. 2001 Mar-Apr;(2):46-9

[7] Journal of Traditional Chinese Medicine 1990 June;10(2):97-8
Ulmus macrocarpa for the treatment of ulcerative colitis--a report of 36 cases
by, Ye G, Cao Q, Chen X, Li S, Jia B.

[8] Pharmacology of Curcuma longa. Planta Med. 1991 Feb;57(1):1-7

Bibliography

Deschauer, Thomas. Complete Course in Herbalism. Self-published. 1940

Nowell, H. Undergraduate Course. Vancouver; Dominion Herbal College, 1926

Walker, N.W. Fresh Vegetable and Fruit Juices. Revised edition, Prescott, Az. Norwalk, 1978

Jethro Kloss, Back to Eden, Back to Eden Books Publishing Company, Loma Linda CA.

Resources:

Water Distillers

Wholesale Water Distillers carries various low cost distillers.
740-544-5842
www.wholesalewaterdistillers.com

Pure Water Inc.
800-875-5915
www.purewaterinc.com

Rebounder

The cellerciser isn't a normal rebounder or mini tramp, its tapered springs allow the body to bounce up and down with low impact on the knees and spine.
800-856-4863
www.cellercise.com

Herbal Education

The School of Natural Healing offers beginning, intermediate, and advanced training in herbology. The School also offers correspondence courses in Aromatherapy, Iridology, and Reflexology.
800-372-8255
www.snh.cc

Dr. Christopher's Publications

The full line of Dr. Christopher's writings are available
800-372-8255
www.snh.cc

Herbs and herbal formulas

Dr. Christopher's Original Formulas are available
888-235-3265
drchristophers.com

Herb Awareness LLC. carries most of the herbal formulas
listed in this book in bulk form.
888-372-4372

Starwest Botainicals carries most herbs in bulk
888-273-4372
starwestherb.com

Horizon Herbs LLC. sells root starts, herb seeds and other herb
growing necessities.
541-846-6704

Juicers

Champion is a reliable name in juicing. Their machine is
strong durable and built to last. Its easy to clean too!
(209)-369-2154
www.championjuicer.com

Slant board

The Williams Company makes a slant board that is cushioned,
folds in two, and is portable.
805-646-9713
www.slant6.com

Index

A

B

D

dairy 86
dandelion 16, 17
defecation 18
dehydrated 32
dehydration 25
demulcent 88
depression 83
destended transverse colon 74
diabetes 25, 46
diarrhea 19, 34, 48, 52, 72
digestive juices 17
digestive system 54
digestives 16
distended abdomen 48
distilled water 40, 73
diverticula 74
diverticular disease 5
diverticulitis 5, 73
Dr. Christopher 4
Dr. Christopher's Publications 92
Dr. John Harvey Kellogg 4, 22, 41
Dr. Nowell 4, 6
Dr. Samuel Thomson 57
duodenum 16
dyspepsia 72, 76

E

Ebers Papyrus 5
eczema 82
elder 14
elimination 20
enema 32, 40
enzyme rich foods 89
enzymes 12, 48, 89
esophagus 14
Essene 6
exercise 40

F

false sweet flag root 14
fecal 31, 34, 59
feces 18

Fen-LB 58
fennel 16, 62
fermented foods 90
fibrous foods 89
fissures 73
fistulas 73
flatulence 75
flax 45
fruits 44

G

gall bladder 16, 53
gall stones 36
garlic 48
garlic implant 44
gas 75
gastric juices 14
Gastro-Intestinal Formula 55
gentian 16
GERD 79
ginger 14, 45, 60
gluten-sensitive 69
golden seal 61

H

halitosis 31
hcl 14
healthy colon 74
heart disease 83
heartburn 76, 79
hemorrhoids 75
hepatic tonics 17
herbal education 92
herbal gruel 45
Herbal LB 58
herbs and herbal formulas 92
hiatal hernia 79
high cholesterol 83
Hindu Vedas 5
Hippocrates 4, 5
honey 36, 44
hormonal problems 83
horseback riding 43
horsemint 16

hydrangea 14
hydrochloric acid 14

I

IBS 77
ileitis 71
ileocecal valve 18
Immucalm 45
indian apple 17
indigestion 76
infertility 83
inflammatory bowel disease 5
insulin 16
intestinal 31, 32
Intestinal Sweeper 46
intrinsic factor 14
irritable bowel syndrome 77

J

jaborandi 14
Jethro Kloss 6
John Harvey Kellogg 6
juicers 93
juices 46

K

Kid-e-Col 38
Kid-E-Reg 57
kimchi 52

L

leaky gut syndrome 77
lemon 14
LES 79
licorice 45, 55
liver 16, 53
liverwort 17
lobelia 45, 57
lovage 16
Lower Bowel Formula 34, 35, 58, 59, 62, 72

M

malnourishment 83

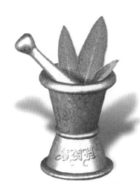

Dr. Christopher's
The School of Natural Healing

College of Herbal Studies

Outstanding Education Since 1953

Herbal Education

The School of Natural Healing was founded in 1953 by Dr. John R. Christopher and has been the means for thousands of students to begin and further their herbal knowledge and wisdom.

Few things are as rewarding and satisfying as being able to care for your own and your family's health. There is no safer avenue than herbal and natural healing, yet many people become overwhelmed at the prospect of herbal study towards becoming their own healer.

The School of Natural Healing's Master Herbalist Program will show you that you can become your own doctor, and that it is not as difficult as you may think. In as little as an hour a day, you could become a qualified healer and teacher in less than two years—all in the comfort of your own home.

Our courses are designed to teach herbalism from the ground up, beginning with foundational understandings of natural methodologies, and progressing through the many aspects of herbal healing, including herb identification, horticulture, medicinal usages, methods of preparation, and more. Students who complete the Master Herbalist Program are prepared to take care of both themselves and their families, and to share their knowledge and wisdom in the service of educating others.

Our School curriculum and philosophy is built upon the understanding and practice of four fundamental principles.

1. **Preventative Nutrition**
2. **Eradicating the Cause of Disease**
3. **Healing the Body through Natural Methods**
4. **Education**

Whether your interest is in a particular skill or in certification, The School of Natural Healing has courses to fit your needs

The Family Herbalist Program (Level 100)

The School's Family Herbalist Course is designed to empower you with the knowledge and confidence needed to tackle almost any health issue. The Family Herbalist Course is essential for anyone who wants to take charge of their own health and become more informed, educated, and independent. This course explores important concepts in natural medicine that even the most experienced natural healers need to know for success.

The Nutritional Herbalist Program (Levels 200-500)

The Nutritional Herbologist Program will instruct you to recognize, understand, and assist the body's inherent healing power. You will learn preventative medicine through the study of basic principles of natural healing. These courses focus on cause of disease, nutrition, elimination therapies, and herbal cleansing for the entire system. Training also includes the proper application of wholesome herbs and simple therapies. Using Dr. Christopher's world-famous herbal combinations and single herbs, you will learn how to cleanse, nourish, and build the body. Prerequisite: Family Herbalist Program

The Herbalist Program (Levels 600-1300)

In the Herbalist Program you will build upon the Nutritional Herbologist training with in-depth instruction in the use of herbal therapy to remove the cause of disease. Within these courses you help fulfill The School's mission to see a competent natural healer in every home. You will learn how to use the natural medicines that surround you with regional materials. In this program you will learn herb identification, selection, harvesting, horticulture, usage, herbal formulation and preparation. With enough materials to create your own herbal library, this program includes 18 hours of herbal therapy instruction from Dr. Christopher himself. A certificate of "Herbalist" is awarded upon completion of the first thirteen levels of the home study program.

The Advanced Hebalist Program (Levels 1400-2200)

The final nine courses of the Master Herbalist Program give you the skills to become a qualified teacher of herbology. As more people seek natural health, the need for competent educators increases in a variety of health related areas. The Advanced Herbalist Program provides the training to place you on the highest level of herbal competency. As a Master Herbalist you can teach others, so that they are able to take responsibility for their own health. The course study and preliminary examinations are administered through correspondence and provide instruction from the highest-qualified herbal practitioners and herbal pharmacists in the field. The final examinations are only administered at the Master Herbalist Certification Seminar, held at our facilities. This seminar gives you the opportunity of fine-tuning your skills with the clinical experience of some of the best herbalists in the country.

Help By Phone

Herbalists and Master Herbalists are available to students for tutorial and study aid by toll-free phone from 10:00 am to 4:00 pm MT Monday - Friday (1-800-372-8255). Master Herbalist David Christopher accepts calls from the general public Monday—Thursday between 1:00 pm and 2:00 pm MT. These calls are limited to 3 minutes each and are for educational instruction only.

Other Services

The School of Natural Healing provides a number of additional educational services and courses:

- Iridology Home Study Courses with David J. Pesek, Ph.D.
- Reflexology Courses
- Aromatherapy Courses
- Seminars with SNH instructors and Master Herbalists in your area.
- Monthly subscriptions to *A Healthier You* Audio Newsletter.
- Texts available on CD Rom for Windows.

For information on any of these services, please call or write to:

The School of Natural Healing
P.O. Box 412   Springville, Utah 84663
1-800-372-8255
www.snh.cc   registration@snh.cc

Dr. Christopher's School of Natural Healing Presents
The Aromatherapy Home Study Program

The art and science of aromatherapy has been practiced for thousands of years. Aromatherapy uses fragrant oils extracted from aromatic plants to aid the body in healing both physical and emotional trauma. Some of these oils can have a profound effect on mood while others are anti-biotic and anti-inflammatory. Aromatherapy is a fun and exciting way to improve your family's health as well as your own.

The School of Natural Healing's Aromatherapy Course will fill your home with fragrances from around the world. Thirty two bottles of essential oils are included in the course along with details on how to use over ninety others. This one of a kind correspondence also includes, seven text books, four study guides, four videos, and two audio cassettes.

Every aspect of basic aromatherapy is covered as well as detailed information on anatomy, and making simple home remedies with common herbs and spices you probably already have in your home.

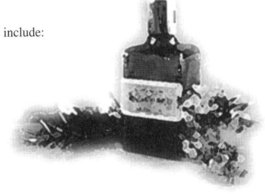

Health problems discussed include:

- headache
- stomachache
- colic
- stress
- hypertension
- foot odor
- skin problems
- infections
- sunburns

This course places special emphasis hands on learning. The student will enjoy making their own essential oil blends and formulas including creams, deodorant, pot-pouri, facial masks, and even perfume or cologne.

Dr. Christopher's School of Natural Healing Presents
Iridology, A Wholistic Approach

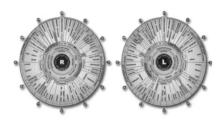

Two Level Iridology Home Study Course & Live Seminar

Dr. John R. Christopher utilized the science of Iridology thoughout his practice, and he had a tremendous appreciation for its benefits and usefulness in assessing health conditions in the body.

The School of Natural Healing has offered iridology study in the past with various teachers, however, in becoming acquainted with Dr. David J. Pesek, we found his understanding and methodology to be the foremost among his contemporaries. Though the mutual cooperation of Dr. Pesek and The School of Natural Healing, we know that we are offering the most comprehensive Iridology course available in North America.

This comprehensive, two level home study program and live seminar offers a fully informative and detailed look at the science and practice of Iridology. Beginning at basic levels and moving forward to advanced understandings of this art and science, the student will gain a powerful knowledge of revealing levels of health, inflammation and degeneration within the human body, along with thought and emotional patterns.

Call now to find out more about this amazing science.

The School of Natural Healing
1-800-372-8255

Dr. Christopher's School of Natural Healing Presents

Reflexology Home Study Program

The School of Natural Healing's Reflexology Home Study Program helps you develop the powerful tools needed to assess health conditions and stimulate the body to heal itself. Reflexology is the study of reflex points found throughout the body and how they can be used to enhance health. Once you understand the basics, your own two hands will be the tools you use to help yourself and your family on the road to great health.

Learn how to deal with any health problem without the side effects of chemical medication. Diseases discussed include:

Heart Disease
Arthritis
Sciatic Pains
Back Problems
Sinus Infections
Diabetes
Kidney Stones
and more

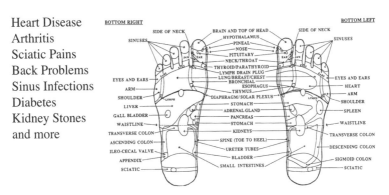

Students of the Reflexology course also receive instruction in basic herbology, anatomy, and physiology. In order to practice reflexology as a profession in most states, one must be a licensed massage therapist. The purpose of this reflexology course is to prepare you to practice reflexology on your family members and yourself without charging for your services. The certificate awarded after completing this course does not entitle you to practice reflexology professionally, teach reflexology, or use the title reflexologist in ads or endorsements. In most states licensed massage therapists may use the title reflexologist after taking this course, state laws may vary.

The School of Natural Healing
1-800-372-8255

CHRISTOPHER ⬤ PUBLICATIONS

P.O. Box 412 · Springville, Utah 84663 1-800-372-8255 · www.snh.cc

Books for your Health and Well-Being

Dr. Christopher's Herbal Seminar Videos (8 VHS video cassettes)

Now available to the public! Over 16 hours of Dr. Christopher on VHS video cassette. Witness America's premier natural healer sharing his knowledge and philosophies gained through years of experience.
Item #99100 $395.00

School of Natural Healing Revised Edition

This monumental work groups herbs by therapeutic action, and treats in great detail their usage and action. A majority of the thousands of herbal formulas used by Dr. Christopher can be found in this book. Also discussed are diseases, their symptoms and causes, and case histories. This new edition contains Dr. Christopher's biography, expanded index, improved format, and updated research.
Item #99101 $39.95

Dr. Christopher's Herb Lectures (10 Compact Discs)

Listen and glean from the knowledge, wit and wisdom of Dr. Christopher teaching the benefits of herbs and natural healing.
Item #99102 $69.95

Every Woman's Herbal

The wisdom of Dr. Christopher combined with the practicality of Cathy Gileadi for the health of women of all ages. 242 pages
Item #99110 $14.95

Herbal Home Health Care

This volume from Dr. Christopher effectively deals with over 50 common ailments, listing the diseases in convenient alphabetical order with concise definitions, symptom descriptions, causes, herbal aids and other natural treatments. 196 pages
Item #99103 $12.95

Dr. Christopher's 3 Day Cleanse, Mucusless Diet and Herbal Combinations
Juice cleansing for detoxification, wholesome diet for health.
Item #99104 $2.00

The Cold Sheet Treatment
Dr. Christopher explains step by step his time-tested treatment for colds, flus, and any feverous or viral condition.
Item #99107 $2.00

Curing the Incurables
Treatment program for conditions deemed "incurable." Dr. Christopher shows "there are no incurable diseases."
Item #99108 $2.00

An Herbal Legacy of Courage by David W. Christopher, M.H.
The first biography of Dr. Christopher. Learn about his youth, his roots in herbalism, and his joys and struggles as he sought to heal and educate all who would hear.
Item #99112 $5.00

For a full publication list, please call or write to:

Christopher Publications
P.O. Box 412   Springville, Utah 84663
1-801-372-8255
of visit our website www.snh.cc

The Complete Herbal Writings of
Dr. John R. Christopher
on CD Rom for Windows

Includes the full texts of:
> School of Natural Healing
> Every Woman's Herbal
> Herbal Home Health Care
> Over 6 years of Dr. Christopher's Newsletters
> Over 2,000 pages of previously unpublished writings

Also includes color pictures of nearly 100 herbs

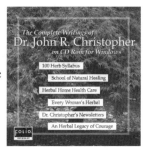

This Folio® based program can allow you to search quickly and easily for any word or topic Dr. Christopher ever wrote about. Search in a particular book or scan the entire library. This easy-to-use CD Rom will speed up your study and research time. (Windows Only)

Only $98.95

A Healthier You Audio Newsletter
1 Year Subscription

These informative audio cassettes are select recordings of Master Herbalist David Christopher's popular radio program "A Healthier You." Each 60 minute cassette offers up-to-date information and common sense regarding a variety of health topics, herbs, natural treatments and therapies.

Only $39.95
Audio Newsletter Back-Issues Available
Look for our list of back-issue titles of cassettes. Single tapes or volumes of 12 are available.

Dr. Christopher's
Natural Healing Newsletters
Back - Issues

Begun as a monthly newsletter in 1980, these various treatises are available in single issuses and in volumes of 12.

Volume 1 Nos. 1 - 12　item #95150
Volume 2 Nos. 1 - 12　item #95250
Volume 3 Nos. 1 - 12　item #95350
Volume 4 Nos. 1 - 12　item #95450
Volume 5 Nos. 1 - 12　item #95550
Volume 6 Nos. 1 - 12　item #95650

Herbal Facts
Information
Case Histories
Recipes
Testimonials
Formulas
and More!